W9-CDP-854

stopping cancer
before it starts

stoppingcancer
before it starts

THE AMERICAN INSTITUTE FOR CANCER RESEARCH'S
PROGRAM FOR CANCER PREVENTION

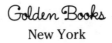

Golden Books
New York

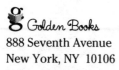
Golden Books

888 Seventh Avenue
New York, NY 10106

Copyright © 1999 by the American Institute for Cancer Research
All rights reserved, including the right of reproduction
in whole or in part in any form.
Golden Books® and colophon
are trademarks of Golden Books Publishing Co., Inc.

The information contained in this book is not intended to be a substitute
for professional medical advice. The reader is advised to consult a physician who can discuss individual needs and provide individual counseling
regarding symptoms and treatment.

Designed by Meryl Sussman Levavi/digitext, inc.

Manufactured in the United States of America

10 9 8 7 6 5 4 3 2 1

Library of Congress Cataloging-in-Publication Data

Stopping cancer before it starts: the AICR program for cancer
    prevention/American Institute for Cancer Research.
        p. cm.
    Includes index.
    ISBN 1-58238-000-7 (hc : alk. paper)
    1. Cancer—Prevention. I. American Institute for Cancer
Research
RC268.S76 1999
616.99'4052—DC21

                                                                 98-24679
                                                                    CIP

contents

part IV

recipes and menus

preface

Since 1983 the American Institute for Cancer Research (AICR) has been at the forefront of the diet, nutrition, and cancer issue. We have seen many changes in that time. In its earliest days, for example, the Institute sometimes found itself attacked by commercial interests for daring to claim that actions as simple as moving to a diet lower in fat and richer in fruits, vegetables, and grains could do something as dramatic as reduce cancer risk. Today, that's a finding that most people accept without question, that many segments of the food industry have found to be a valuable marketing approach, and that is backed by a wealth of scientific data.

But reaching that point has not come easily. AICR is a pioneer in building public awareness of the role of diet and nutrition in the prevention of cancer with extensive national consumer education programs. The Institute has also funded tens of millions of dollars for research in diet, nutrition, and cancer, helping scientists better understand the link between the foods we choose and cancer prevention. And yet we are well aware that there is still much more to be done, both in research related to diet, nutrition and cancer, and in educating consumers to make effective changes for cancer prevention. Reaching consumers is one reason for this book, and for the landmark scientific report upon which it is based.

The Institute's efforts in cancer research and education reached a new peak with the beginning of the Diet and Cancer Project several years ago and the recent production and publication of that project's major report, *Food, Nutrition and the Prevention of Cancer: A Global Perspective*. This international report is the result of more than four years of work by the staff of AICR and its international affiliate, the World Cancer Research Funds (WCRF), the dedication and efforts of an expert panel of fifteen of the world's leading scientists in diet and cancer, and the contributions of more than one hundred

1

other scientists and policy markers from around the world. It is a report that is helping set new directions in cancer research and public health policy around the world. It is also the foundation for this book.

Food, Nutrition and the Prevention of Cancer: A Global Perspective was created primarily for researchers, health professionals, and those involved in forming public health policy. Yet its scientific findings, cancer prevention recommendations, and the new understanding of the cancer process presented in its pages also have much to offer the average consumer. Bringing that information to the you, the consumer, in an understandable and usable form is the reason for this book.

Stopping Cancer Before It Starts was created to help you understand the cancer process, to present some of the most important science behind the new recommendations to prevent cancer, and to provide you with practical tools to help you make changes to lower cancer risk.

What's important here is not whether you follow all the science presented or try all the recipes offered. What really matters is that you realize that cancer can be prevented and that your actions play a vital role in making lower cancer risk a reality for you and your family. The message throughout this book is a simple one—there are things you can do today to reduce your risk of cancer. Not quick fixes but basic lifestyle and dietary changes that will mean lower cancer risk for life.

It is our hope that what is offered here will change your life in a positive and more healthful way. Working together, we can make cancer prevention a reality.

MARILYN GENTRY
President, American Institute for Cancer Research

introduction

Why this book?

Because cancer can be prevented!

For several years, the research community has been aware that cancer is a disease over which we have a surprising amount of control. That awareness is now growing among consumers, and it is the aim of the American Institute for Cancer Research (AICR) to make it grow further. Breakthroughs in research and treatment procedures have brought dramatic increases in survival rates for many forms of cancer. These breakthroughs indicate that cancer is not a mysterious disease about which we can do little or nothing. And now there is even more reason for hope. Why?

Because cancer can be prevented!

A growing body of scientific evidence clearly shows that most cancers can be prevented, not through new medical breakthroughs or miracle drugs, but simply through the way we live. Researchers now estimate that 60 percent to 70 percent of all cancers are directly linked to the foods we eat and related lifestyle factors, including smoking, exercise, and obesity. The federal government's National Cancer Institute reports that as many as 35 percent of cancer deaths are diet-related. If you add to that those that are related to smoking and alcohol, as many as three-quarters of all cancer deaths are diet- or lifestyle-related.

Since 1983 AICR has made cancer prevention one of its primary objectives. While AICR has been one of the primary funding sources for research in the areas of diet, nutrition, and cancer, it has also been the leading source of consumer-oriented educational materials about diet, nutrition, and reducing cancer risk.

Now there is even stronger evidence that we can take concrete action to dramatically reduce our cancer risk. In 1994 AICR, in collaboration with its affiliate in the United Kingdom, the World Cancer Research Fund (WCRF), launched the Diet and Cancer Project. The purpose of this effort was to provide a detailed review of the thousands of research projects in diet and cancer that had been undertaken over the past decade and to develop new recommendations for cancer prevention.

The project was spearheaded by an expert panel of many of the leading researchers from around the world. In addition, it involved more than a hundred scientists as contributors and peer reviewers. Also contributing to the project as participating observers were representatives from the World Health Organization (WHO), the International Agency for Research on Cancer (IARC), the Food and Agriculture Organization (FAO) of the United Nations, and the U.S. government's National Cancer Institute (NCI).

More than forty-five hundred research projects were reviewed as part of the Diet and Cancer Project. In addition, a series of international review meetings were held, allowing for discussion of the materials being evaluated, input by local scientists from different parts of the world, and the development of new recommendations and guidelines. The culmination of this effort came in October of 1997 with the publication of *Food, Nutrition and the Prevention of Cancer: A Global Perspective.* Targeted at scientists and those involved in public health policy, this report provided the most comprehensive review of research in diet and cancer to date, and was the first to examine diet and cancer prevention from an international point of view. This information is now in the hands of more than 30,000 scientists and public-policy makers around the world, and is helping to direct research efforts and shape policy decisions related to cancer and its prevention.

Stopping Cancer Before It Starts takes the research and recommendations contained in *Food, Nutrition and the Prevention of Cancer* and presents them in a format that is highly readable and understandable. But most important of all, it presents them in a way that is highly practical, offering concrete and often quite simple ways that you—today—can reduce your own risk of cancer.

While newspaper headlines about research on cancers linked to our genes may grab a great deal of attention, the real news is that the vast majority of cancers can be prevented. The primary causes of cancer in this country aren't genetics, pollution, pesticides, or any of the many other things the media promotes as the latest "cancer scare." What you'll learn in this book is that while the causes of cancer may surround us daily, the means to prevent those cancers also surround us.

Stopping Cancer Before It Starts is a practical handbook—one that helps you to understand cancer as a disease, that empowers you, and that enables you to lower your cancer risk as much as possible. This book provides a basic explanation of the cancer process in clear, understandable terms: what causes cancer, why we get cancer, and what happens within our bodies that can make us fall victim to this disease—or not. And while that's all information worth knowing, the real value of this book is in the actions it recommends you take, starting today. You may have heard some of these recommendations before, perhaps in confusing, incomplete, or sometimes contradictory reports in the media. But here, we will clarify that information for you and add a lot of new information that you likely don't already know. *Stopping Cancer Before It Starts* gives you a comprehensive plan for cancer prevention. Here you'll find a wide variety of current, reliable, scientifically proven advice, all integrated into a practical plan for healthy living and cancer prevention. *Stopping Cancer Before It Starts* doesn't offer a quick fix that will cure cancer or somehow make you cancer-proof. What it does offer is the next-best thing, an achievable approach to nutrition and lifestyle that not only reduces cancer risk but also leads to reduced risk for heart disease, diabetes, obesity, and many other chronic health problems.

You'll find suggestions on how to get more physical activity into your life, on how to make healthier food choices, and on how to make a variety of small changes in how you live. These often minor, incremental changes add up to a big change in your overall health. You'll also find a recipe section that clearly illustrates how interesting, exciting, and delicious eating for better health and lower cancer risk can be.

This book will empower you. The first thing it makes clear is that cancer, in the vast majority of cases, is not something that simply "happens." Yes, everyone is a candidate to get cancer. This is simply a biological fact of the cells that make up our bodies. But at the same time, nearly everyone is a candidate *not* to get cancer.

All of us can take actions that, in the vast majority of cases, help enable our bodies to strengthen their natural protective mechanisms against the potential cancer-causing agents we live with every day.

Yes, this is a book that will ask you to look at your life and perhaps make a variety of changes. It will ask you to think differently about the foods you select. It will ask you to act differently in regard to exercise and watching your weight. It will ask you to take action, to do things now so that cancer doesn't strike sometime in an uncertain future.

Most of us are used to being rewarded rather quickly for the positive actions we take, and usually we expect those rewards almost immediately—we make that big sale and get a bonus; we lose twenty pounds and suddenly start getting compliments. This book, on the other hand, will tell you how you can do things to help ensure that, in effect, "nothing" happens—that five, ten, or maybe twenty, thirty, forty years or more in the future, cancer is a disease you simply won't have to face.

That may be a long time for many people to wait for nothing to happen. Is it worth it? That's a bit like asking, "Is it worth saving for retirement?" If you've ever known anyone who has suffered through cancer, including those who have successfully been through surgery, chemotherapy, and recovery, you already know the answer to that question. Virtually anything we can do to help ensure that cancer doesn't strike is worth it.

This book won't ask you to do anything that requires dramatic changes in your life or that requires missing out on things you enjoy and value. The advice offered here is for positive actions that are easy to accomplish and that supply both short- and long-term benefits.

While cancer prevention may be the ultimate goal of the advice offered in this book, the overall health consequences of following that advice are significant and much more immediate. Follow this book's recommendations on food choices and physical activity, and you'll probably find that you have more energy, that you're more fit, and that you've become a much trimmer you. You should find that you have a better attitude about most things related to your health. You should learn a good deal about cancer that you didn't know—and, we hope, you'll have a new opinion about what cancer is and what you can do about it.

There is, of course, no guarantee when it comes to cancer. While our knowledge of this disease has increased dramatically over the past two decades, we still know too little to ensure that cancer will never strike any one individual. But we do know more than enough to change the odds and change them dramatically.

The term *cancer prevention* is often used today to mean preventing someone from dying of this disease—usually through earlier detection and effective treatment. While that certainly is a much desired goal, our objective through the Diet and Cancer Project, through this book, and through AICR's ongoing programs is crystal clear—to do all we can to help people make sure that cancer never strikes at all. What this book offers is the best advice currently available for cancer prevention in its best and most basic form—stopping cancer before it starts. It is our hope that this book can help make that goal a reality for you.

part I

*what you need to
know about cancer*

1

before we begin: separating the facts from myths about cancer

This isn't a "diet" book in any conventional sense. It is not the "Anti-Cancer Diet." There can be no such thing. Still, the research is clear: You can eat your way to good health as long as you know which kinds of foods are going to promote good health, which are not, and how to integrate them with an active lifestyle.

Before we get down to the basic mechanics of cancer—how it starts and how the body thwarts it with its numerous defense mechanisms (many of them enhanced—or diminished—by diet)— right now let's clear up a few of the myths that persist about cancer, what it is, and who is likely to get it.

The figure on the following page is a pie graph that illustrates the percentages of all cancers and their roots in different known risk factors.[1] Because it is impossible to know the precise origin of *every* cancer, the figures are of necessity averages. (Many cancers, as we shall explore, are probably caused by the intersection of more than one risk factor—it is difficult, for example, to sort out whether a particular cancer is caused by a sedentary lifestyle or obesity, two risk factors that often go hand in hand.)

---

[1] SOURCE: *The Harvard Report on Cancer Prevention.*

That approximately 30 percent of all cancers are tobacco-related will probably surprise no one. But that overall lifestyle factors, including tobacco use, diet, and exercise, are at the root of more than three-quarters of all cancers is eye-opening. We all know that obesity and eating "heart attack foods" can result in heart disease, diabetes, and other chronic illness, but how many of us were aware that these lifestyle factors are also at the root of most cancers? If you worry more about prolonged exposure to sunlight (ultraviolet radiation) than you do about eating fatty or processed foods, you may be surprised to note that the overeating of such foods is probably at the root of fifteen times more cancers than *all* types of radiation.

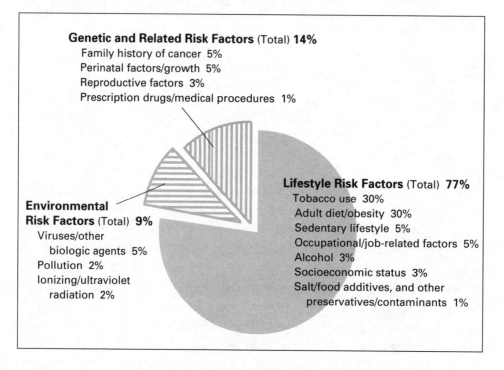

Genetic and Related Risk Factors (Total) **14%**
  Family history of cancer 5%
  Perinatal factors/growth 5%
  Reproductive factors 3%
  Prescription drugs/medical procedures 1%

Environmental Risk Factors (Total) **9%**
  Viruses/other
    biologic agents 5%
  Pollution 2%
  Ionizing/ultraviolet
    radiation 2%

Lifestyle Risk Factors (Total) **77%**
  Tobacco use 30%
  Adult diet/obesity 30%
  Sedentary lifestyle 5%
  Occupational/job-related factors 5%
  Alcohol 3%
  Socioeconomic status 3%
  Salt/food additives, and other
    preservatives/contaminants 1%

In order to talk about cancer more sensibly, let's clear up right now some of the common misconceptions about what cancer is and is not.

myth: Cancer is a single disease.

fact: Cancer is actually more than a hundred different diseases with one thing in common: genetic mutations. These genetic mutations can take place in several different ways, as we shall discuss in chapter 2, but most of them are due to lifestyle and dietary factors.

myth: Exposure to a single carcinogen (cancer-causing agent) causes cancer.

fact: We are exposed to potential carcinogens all the time (just as we are exposed to bacteria and viruses all the time). Each of our some 10 trillion cells takes approximately 10,000 "hits" every day from one or another potentially mutating agent, and for the most part, cancer on the cellular level is a comparatively rare phenomenon. It is most often chronic, long-term exposure to carcinogens—usually coupled with diet- or lifestyle-related diminishment in our built-in cancer defenses—that results in cancer. As noted above, our bodies are equipped with an array of cancer-fighting defense mechanisms (see "Our Defense Mechanisms" in chapter 3) that are "designed" to prevent potential mutations and root out mutations that do take place.

myth: Cancer just happens.

fact: Carcinogenesis, or the cancer process (literally, from the Latin *birth* or *origin, of the crab*), is a long-term or chronic process, sometimes taking as many as two or three or four decades to produce cancer, just as cardiovascular disease is a process, which, after a few decades, can produce veins so clogged that a stroke or heart attack results. Certain carcinogens are so powerful that they can shorten the decades-long process, but these account for a very few cancers overall.

myth: Whether or not I'll get cancer is built into my genes and there's nothing I can do about it.

fact: While cancer is a genetic disease in the sense that its root is a genetic mutation or a series of genetic mutations, the vast majority of cancers are not inherited. While genetics is an important tool in cancer research, prevention, and treatment, in certain respects news of genetic research increases many of the public's misconceptions about cancer. Because of the discovery of genes linked to certain cancers, many take the understandable but incorrect view that "If it's in my genes, then there's nothing I can do about it."

We are here to tell you that genes are by no means destiny. It is increasingly clear that, for most of us, much of our cancer destiny is in our own hands.

To illustrate the equation of genetics and lifestyle, think of it this way: If you're fair-skinned (a genetic predisposition), you're much more likely to get a bad sunburn (lifestyle/environment) than someone with dark skin. This could, in turn, lead to an increased likelihood of skin cancer. However, if you never allow yourself to be roasted on the beach, your risk of skin cancer will probably be quite low, despite having an acknowledged risk factor. With very few exceptions, cancers that are believed to be genetically linked are also strongly linked to diet, nutrition, and lifestyle, and thus potentially capable of being prevented through such means.

Despite genetic links, there is most definitely something you can do about reducing cancer risk. In reality, the genetic link has more to do with how your body deals with the insults to which it's exposed. Your lifestyle choices can play a major role in countering increased risk due to your genetics.

myth: Women in my family have had breast cancer, so I'm at greater risk for developing breast cancer.

fact: While there is some connection between breast cancer and genes, even those who have tested positive for the "breast cancer gene" (known as BRCA) are not guaranteed to get cancer. While testing positive for BRCA1 or BRCA2 may indicate a higher risk factor, lifestyle and dietary factors are much more likely to play a role in increased or decreased cancer risk.

myth: Environmental pollution and toxins, such as pesticides and food colorings and other food additives, cause a large percentage of cancers.

fact: There is no good evidence to support the notion that environmental toxins such as pesticides or industrial waste account for any more than a very slight percentage (2 to 5 percent) of all cancers. If you happen to have spent your formative years on Love Canal or next to a toxic dump, then your risk may be considerably different. There is no reliable evidence *at all* that food additives (colorings, preservatives, and so on), contaminants (such as chemicals that may leach out of plastic wraps), and pesticides, when used according to federal regulations, account for any notable increase in cancer risk. In many respects, as we shall explore as we go along, it is more likely that the foods themselves and the quantities of them we eat have much more to do with cancer risk than anything that may be added to them.

myth: Electromagnetic fields, such as those produced by televisions, computer monitors, microwave ovens, and power lines, are a significant cause of cancer.

fact: While it is possible (but by no means conclusively proven) that these factors may cause some cancers, compared to such lifestyle factors as obesity and a sedentary lifestyle, they are pretty close to insignificant for most of us.

myth: Particular foods cause cancer.

fact: While certain foods, certain methods of preparing or preserving foods (such as smoking and salting), and toxins (such as aflatoxin) that can occur in spoiled foods are related to a slightly higher risk of certain kinds of cancers, brief exposure to these potential carcinogens is not likely to lead to cancer. As previously noted, cancer is a chronic process, and it is the repeated and prolonged exposure to these kinds of foods or food preparations that may eventually defeat our defense mechanisms, thus increasing risk of cancer. (Just as there are no guarantees that you *won't* get cancer, there are also no guarantees that you *will*. Even if you smoke, you're more likely to die of heart disease before lung cancer has the chance to strike.) In chapter 7, we will discuss different health aspects of the foods we eat, including how you can create your own cancer-reduction diet. In chapters 8 and 9, we will discuss specific categories of foods and how they affect cancer risk.

myth: Once the cancer initiation process has started, there is nothing I can do to stop it.

fact: The cancer initiation process (see chapter 3) takes place over an extended period of time. The available evidence suggests that there are many ways you can help your body prevent cancer from starting, or stop it in its tracks. This does not mean, however, that if you are diagnosed with cancer, you can cure yourself just by eating right (although you may be able to assist your own treatment and speed your recovery by making dietary and lifestyle changes). It *does* mean that by eating right over the long term, keeping your energy intake and expenditure balanced, and avoiding such lifestyle follies as smoking and heavy drinking, you can keep your defense mechanisms working as they were intended to work and knock out cancer before it occurs. For the most part, all of this will happen without your knowledge—as far as you will *know,* nothing will happen. Your life will go on.

myth: A high percentage of cancers is caused by ultraviolet (sunlight) and ionizing (X rays, gamma rays, etc.) radiation.

fact: While most skin cancers (the majority of which are easily cured if caught early) are caused by ultraviolet radiation, taken together both ionizing and ultraviolet radiation account for only a small number of cancer deaths—about 2 percent. It is true that dietary factors can actually reduce the likelihood of skin cancer in those who have been overexposed to UV radiation, just as dietary factors can reduce the likelihood of cancer in anyone who has been exposed to potential carcinogens.

are we in the midst of a cancer epidemic?

No, but there are worrisome as well as promising statistics.

Mortality rates from cancers across the board rose slightly during the forty-year period between 1950 and 1990, although almost all of that rise can be attributed to lung cancer. If you remove lung cancer from the equation, mortality from cancers is actually down approximately 15 percent during that period, according to American Cancer Society statistics.

Given the amount of research done and the advancements made in cancer treatment, you might think that mortality (deaths) from cancer should have declined steadily. Why hasn't this happened?

There are many reasons, probably many more than can be sensibly enumerated here. The most prominent of these, however, is that we live longer.

Given that the process of carcinogenesis often requires as many as several decades before it results in the event of cancer, someone who in 1951 might have died in an automobile accident (no seat belts or air bags) or from heart disease (no transplants or bypass surgery), might in 1991 live long enough for the cancer odds to catch up. But if cancer isn't inevitable, why should living longer make a difference?

It makes a difference because of the statistics: We all have to die of something. We've been remarkably successful at reducing the incidence of a lot of those other somethings, so given that we all have to go somehow, as one mortality rate falls another will automatically rise. This does not mean that you will get cancer automatically when you get old. Cardiovascular disease is still the number one killer of Americans. There are, however, a number of researchers who believe that simply through dietary, nutritional, and lifestyle means we may be able to extend our life expectancy by many years. What's good for beating cancer is also good for beating many other chronic diseases.

Consider smoking, and again consider that cancers can take two, three, or more decades to appear: while many Americans have stopped smoking, those who may have smoked during the glamour days of the cigarette—the 1940s through 1970s—may only now or in the last two decades be developing tobacco-related cancers. In the next thirty to forty years, if the incidence of smoking among Americans continues to decline, so should the incidence of cancer, particularly lung cancer, associated with tobacco. The same is true of cancers linked to diet. Those who were busy consuming what we often think of as "heart-attack foods" or drinking more heavily during that same time frame, may only have begun, in the last couple of decades, to see the results of these choices.

a short history of cancer

Cancer is by no means a modern illness, although some have called it the disease of urbanization and industrialization. Evidence of cancer has been found dating back to the dawn of time, in fossils of animals and in mummified human remains.

The word *cancer* comes from the Latin for *crab,* and its first recorded use is by the legendary Greek physician Hippocrates, around 400 B.C. Hippocrates described in his writings diseases that were probably cancers of the stomach, rectum, breast, uterus, and many other tissues.

Hippocrates and other early physicians knew nothing about cells, but understood that some abnormal growths were benign, or self-limiting, and others were malignant, which, crablike, continued to claw their way through the body, gobbling up everything in their paths until the host, or victim, died.

Cells were first seen by human eyes in 1665 when scientist Robert Hooke examined a piece of cork under one of the earliest microscopes. He named the individual chambers he saw in the cork *cells* because they reminded him of the distinct and separate cells of a jail. Famed Dutch scientist

Antonie van Leeuwenhoek was the first to describe living cells a few years later, but it took two more centuries for scientists to develop optics sophisticated enough to map cells and gather a more thorough understanding of what cells do.

Aided by microscopes, these later physicians understood that cancer was a disease of the cells. In the nineteenth century, German physiologist Johannes Müller noted that the cells in cancerous tumors appeared to be quite different from normal cells. He found that they were as hungry and rapidly growing as those found in developing embryos.

Although cancer has always been with us—as noted previously, it appears to be the price we pay for our remarkable adaptability—it's impossible to know what the incidence of cancer was in early humans. Some have maintained that cancer was rare among hunter–gatherer and pastoral peoples living in remote parts of the world, such as the Himalayas, the Arctic, and equatorial Africa, when first visited by European explorers. Many have taken these sorts of reports to indicate that our preagricultural ancestors probably didn't have a very high incidence of cancer, either. Some have extended this even further to suggest that cancer is a disease of civilization.

Much of this will have to remain speculation: There simply is no adequate record to calculate. If early humans did not get cancer, it may be simply because they did not live long enough.

But there is another possible explanation: If indeed those of our hunter–gatherer ancestors who lived long lives did not experience rates of cancer equivalent to today's, it would most likely have been due to diet and high levels of physical activity. Their diets would have included high levels of fresh vegetables and fruits, next-to-no consumption of simple sugars, and very low levels of saturated fats. The meat they ate would have come from wild animals who were themselves quite lean and fed on fresh fruits and vegetables, or on other lean animals. Because our hunting and gathering ancestors would have had to hunt and gather their food, obesity would have been rare—it's hard to get fat when you have to chase breakfast, lunch, *and* dinner.

Also important is the issue of detection and the explosion of knowledge in the last ten to fifteen years. Look at any book or a brochure about cancer from as recently as five years ago and you'll probably find a list of the "warning signs of cancer." These signs are still valid and useful today—changes in bowel habits, lumps, sores that won't heal, and so on—yet they are a good example of how far our understanding of cancer and our ability to detect it have come in such a short time. These warning signs are symptoms of disease that's already passed through initiation and promotion, and into the progression stage (see "How Cancer Happens and How Our Bodies Thwart It" in chapter 2). With self-exams, pap smears, blood tests, magnetic resonance imaging, antigen and genetic testing, and still other means, we can detect cancers of all sorts much earlier than ever before—and in the past many of these may never have been detected at all. If someone in his eighties with heart disease tests positive for prostate cancer, the chances are that the heart disease will take his life before the cancer has a chance to progress. Before a sophisticated test like the PSA, or prostate-specific antigen (which has led to an increased level of diagnosis for prostate cancer), that individual's prostate cancer would not have been detected until the likelihood of successful treatment dropped considerably—and chances for mortality rose proportionately.

Without looking at the statistics, you might think from all the media coverage that breast cancer mortality rates have increased; but in recent years, despite an increase in the incidence of breast cancer, mortality has declined by some 6 percent, according to the Department of Health and Human Services.

The increased incidence of breast cancer (even in men) is a worrisome statistic. Some of the lower incidence of breast cancer forty years ago may be due to underreporting of cases. It may seem remarkable to young women of this day that breast cancer (indeed, cancer in general) was once seen as shameful and almost taboo, spoken of in hushed tones. Certainly some of the publicity on the increase in incidence may be due to the increase in willingness to talk about the disease. Some of it may be due to better detection. Certainly the decline in mortality is a result of better, earlier treatment. But the picture is far from clear. The increased incidence of breast cancer is probably due to a host of reasons, with many if not most of them related to lifestyle, environment, and diet. The increase in lung cancer rates is proportionate to the increase in smoking among women, and smoking—with its accompanying suppression of the immune system, a poor diet, and decreased levels of physical activity—may lead to physiological conditions that make cancers that are unrelated to smoking more likely.

But there are other culprits to consider. Statistics show that women who reach puberty earlier than normal (eight to nine years of age, rather than twelve to thirteen) have a higher incidence of breast cancer. Indeed, each year that onset of puberty is delayed may confer on a woman as much as a one-fifth reduction in her risk of breast cancer. The problem is that in recent years the average onset of puberty has come earlier and earlier. A century ago, the average age for the onset of menses was fifteen and a half. Today, according to *The Harvard Guide to Women's Health,* the average age is twelve and a half.

Much of this is believed to be due to nutritional and lifestyle factors. High energy diets (lots of protein and simple carbohydrates) and childhood obesity (also on the rise) have been shown to be important factors for early onset of puberty. High levels of physical activity (whether it is involvement in sports or performing chores at home) have been shown to delay onset of puberty. (It's worth noting that studies of boys and girls who reach puberty early or late show that self-esteem for boys rises if they experience early onset of puberty. For girls, however, the opposite is true. Self-esteem tends to fall. Again, however, this may be due to a host of factors, perhaps including those physiological factors that led to early onset of puberty in the first place—obesity, a sedentary lifestyle, and so on. It should be said, however, that either childhood obesity or a sedentary lifestyle during childhood does not automatically lead to early menarche or onset of puberty. Still, they *are* more likely to lead to poorer health in adulthood and increased risk of many diseases, including cancer.)

Other factors to consider in breast cancer are environment and lifestyle. Over the last thirty to forty years, the age at which many women have children has increased. Women who have children before thirty years of age have a lower incidence of breast cancer; women who have children after thirty have a higher risk; and women who never have children have the highest risk. This seems to be due to the differentiation that takes place in breast tissue during the hormonal transformation during a full-term pregnancy. The average woman forty years ago was likely to have more children than a woman today is, and would have begun bearing children at an earlier age, despite what the surge in teenage pregnancies in recent years might lead one to believe. Pregnancy, of course, halts menses, which does not resume again until about eight weeks after delivery in women who do not nurse their babies. In lactating women, periods may not return for several months and may not return immediately after the baby is weaned. Those tissues that cycle in and out of readiness for pregnancy would stay in place for two to as many as several months rather than one. This decrease in the need for uterine lining and other related cells to replicate would naturally reduce the opportunities for the genetic material in these cells to mutate.

Many researchers have theorized that certain industrial toxins at large in the environment have "estrogenic" properties (properties that cause them to mimic the actions of the estrogens our bodies produce, but sometimes much more powerfully). These chemicals may be at the root of the increase in breast cancer—but even so, the increase in risk, if any, is theorized to be comparatively small. A recent study at Harvard University looked at the levels of certain industrial chemicals in a group of five hundred women. All of the women were involved in another long-term study at the university. Half had been diagnosed with breast cancer between 1990 and 1992. The other half were cancer-free. Blood samples from the women had been frozen in 1989. Both groups showed essentially the same levels of two chemicals under investigation—the insecticide DDT and the class of industrial chemicals often associated with toxic waste and known as PCBs (polychlorinated biphenyls). Neither chemical has been produced in this country for the last twenty years but both are still somewhat abundant in the environment. The investigators found the results inconclusive. Other smaller studies have shown a link between levels of the chemicals and incidence of breast cancer. But the fact that the studies are contradictory is itself worrisome. In an editorial that accompanied the report in the *New England Journal of Medicine,* scientist Stephen H. Safe theorized that if there is a link between breast cancer and estrogenic chemicals, it might be offset by antiestrogenic chemicals in food. This study did not, for example, measure the intake of leafy green vegetables in the control group against those in the affected group or the level of physical activity they enjoyed. If it had been able to do so, it might have shown that the cancer-free women's bodies were able to fight off cancer because they had better diets and a more active lifestyle.

From all available evidence, we are not in the midst of a cancer epidemic (any more than we are in the midst of a heart disease epidemic). There are certain types of cancer that are more common in modern, industrialized countries—breast cancer is a case in point—and many of these can be linked directly to nutrition and lifestyle. It is worth noting that of the women who are diagnosed each year, 70 percent have *no* typically recognized risk factor such as the breast cancer gene.

Changes in nutrition and lifestyle (toward a higher energy, lower nutrition "Western" diet) in the developing world have also led to corresponding surges in the same sorts of cancers that plague the industrialized world.

One of the most compelling pieces of evidence that nutritional, environmental, and lifestyle factors profoundly affect cancer risk is that immigrants take on the same cancer risk as that of the natives of their new country—in the *first* generation. Asian women, for example, have a relatively low risk of breast cancer. Women in the United States have some of the highest risk in the world. Upon moving to the United States, Asian women soon assume the same risk as their American neighbors, who have an 11 percent chance of developing the disease within their lifetime and a 3 to 4 percent chance of dying from it.

The World Health Organization reports that about 10 million cancer cases occur worldwide each year, but they estimate that that number will grow to almost 15 million in just the next 20 years, with the majority of growth occurring in the developing nations.

While we may not be in the midst of a cancer epidemic, cancer is and should be a primary health concern of all Americans—too many of whom will die from a disease that can largely be avoided.

2

cancer 101

who will get cancer?

The bad news first: Nearly *anyone* is a candidate for cancer. According to statistics compiled by the American Cancer Society, half of all men and a third of all women in the United States have a lifetime risk of developing some sort of cancer. That's *risk,* not guarantee. If those sound like scary statistics, they are—from a public health perspective. But from the point of view of the individual, they don't need to be scary at all. If they seem to contradict the information contained in the last chapter, they don't really.

Many people have the mistaken notion that cancer, like eye color, is a toss of the genetic dice—some people have blue eyes and some people don't, and there's not much we can do to change it. There are a few very rare genetic combinations that will apparently lead inevitably to cancer. But for the most part, as we shall see, cancer is anything but inevitable.

"Risk" is a number derived from statistical averages and it takes into account *everyone* in *every* kind of lifestyle and all possible cancers over a lifetime (one person may get three). So risk takes into account everyone from AIDS victims, coal miners, asbestos workers, and the most obese, sedentary alcoholic smokers to the most healthy, clean-living, athletic, and diet-conscious among us. It includes exposure to environmental toxins, genetic predisposition, and any other factors you could think of. So if you took a thousand people off the street (or off their couches) and put them all in a room, about half of the men and about a third of the women *might* get cancer sometime during their lifetimes. And then again, maybe not.

It is true that statistics show that about 30 percent of everyone on the planet will "present" (or be diagnosed) with cancer at sometime during their lifetime. That risk is global, and makes the United States cancer risk of 50 percent seem proportionately high. But as it is global, it may not tell us very much about the United States population. Many people around the world simply don't live long enough to get cancer. As cancer is a process that can take decades, the longer people in a given population live, the greater their *statistical* likelihood of getting cancer. Our comparative longevity may increase our risk simply by increasing our length of exposure to carcinogenic compounds.

Think of risk this way: If you're a truck driver and on the road nearly all the time, then your overall *statistical* risk of being involved in an automobile accident is going to be higher than if you're a city dweller who never drives. However, if you're a truck driver who always wears a seat belt, never drives when tired, always obeys speed limits and other traffic laws, always makes sure your rig is in perfect working order, and avoids driving in hazardous conditions, you could avoid all but the most freakish accidents. If you're a drug-abusing truck driver who always speeds and has worn-out tires and brakes, then while your statistical risk of being in an accident may be the same as a safe driver—and while you indeed may never get into an accident—your *actual* risk is going to be considerably higher.

Now the good news, in case you haven't already guessed it: Nearly anyone is also a candidate for *not* getting cancer.

What's clear from the all of the statistics and studies is that cancer risk is a balance, or spectrum, and where you stand in that balance or spectrum—heavily weighted toward high cancer risk, or heavily weighted towards low cancer risk—will depend in large part upon your lifestyle and nutritional choices. And the research suggests that even if you have up until now followed a high-risk lifestyle and nutritional pattern, you can still revise your lifestyle and nutritional practices and reduce your risk.

Risk is a maybe. Cancer risk is a maybe you can do something about.

Eating a cancer-healthy diet and living a cancer-healthy lifestyle are a little like putting on a seat belt and obeying traffic laws—they automatically drop your risk, not only for cancer but for most other chronic diseases.

The guidelines in this book are intended to show you how you can—practically, workably, and sensibly—put yourself on the cancer-healthy side of that risk balance.

what is cancer?

Cancer is a genetic disease in the sense that it can result when our genetic material becomes mutated and the mutation evades the body's cancer prevention system. This cancer prevention system is a fundamental part of the immune system. In the same way that we are exposed to potential infection from bacterial and viral agents almost constantly, and these agents are thwarted by the immune system, so are we constantly exposed to carcinogens. As with viruses and bacteria, most often our bodies quite readily thwart these agents. But our bodies don't do this entirely on their own. It's been known since the early 1950s that particular dietary constituents can actually prevent tumors from forming, even after tissues have been exposed to known carcinogens.

is cancer a rare disease?

On the cellular level, cancer is actually a rare event. You probably know someone who's had cancer, perhaps even several people, so the logical question is, *How can cancer be rare?*

Consider that the adult human body has approximately 10 trillion cells. Consider, also, that a cancer that could spread throughout the whole body begins in just *one* of these cells. Given that it is possible for the DNA in any living cell to mutate and result in cancer, those are pretty astonishing numbers—1 out of 10 trillion. Okay, you say, but people still get cancer—even if only about 30 percent of the world population is ever diagnosed with cancer during their lifetimes, isn't that still nearly a one in three chance?

The answer is both yes and no. Statistically speaking, the answer is yes.

But realistically speaking, the answer is much closer to no. If you refer to the figure on page 10 and rule out the approximately 30 percent of cancers that are related to smoking, and then rule out the much smaller percentage we can't do anything about (inherited genetic disorders, accidental exposure to lethal doses of radiation, skin cancers resulting from overexposure to the sun years ago), then it's clear that you can make your likelihood of getting cancer much lower.

Are you aware that right now, as you read, your body is fighting off cancer on literally thousands of different fronts? If each of our cells is *daily* bombarded about 10,000 times with carcinogenic compounds—many of which are simply by-products of life itself—that's 10 thousand times 10 trillion "hits" per day; and when you consider that out of all of those hits, one cell in 30 percent of people worldwide mutates sufficiently enough to cause cancer, that's an astonishing winning percentage.

But we can do even better. It's possible that by dietary and lifestyle means alone we could reduce that number over time to 20 percent or less of the world population ever getting diagnosed with cancer—and that leaves out tobacco-related cancers entirely. If there are approximately 6 billion people in the world, that's approximately 600 million cases of cancer that could be prevented. *Yours* could be one of those.

If the body is so well-equipped to prevent cancer, why do we get it at all?

Although the full answer is considerably more complex, the simple answer is that cancer is the price we pay for being as adaptable as we are. While genetic mutations can be harmful and cause cancer and other illness, without our genetic mutability we probably wouldn't even exist as a species. The risk of not surviving as individuals is the price we pay to survive as a species.

Understanding how the risky part of genetic mutability occurs gives us the power to make it less risky.

When we do get one of that large number of preventable cancers, it may be in part because we simply have not been aware of how we can help our bodies' plentiful defense mechanisms stop cancers before they start. But to understand how our defense mechanisms work, it helps to understand what cancer is.

Cancer is at least a hundred separate diseases that can affect tissues throughout the body, from the blood to the liver to the brain to the bone. While most cancers are preventable, treatment has improved so much over the last twenty-five years that most cancers are highly curable if caught in their early stages. This is the difference between the *incidence* of cancer and cancer *mortality.* While medicine has reduced mortality, we can on our own reduce incidence, which will automatically reduce mortality—you cannot die of what you do not have.

the birth of the crab: an overview of the cancer process

Carcinogenesis, or the cancer process, translates from the Latin as "birth (or origin) of the crab," and the ancients saw the disease as clawing its way, crablike, through the body, taking over organ after organ, devouring the victim piecemeal. The ancients had no idea why it happened and were helpless to do anything about it. Today we know why and how it happens (although we don't know all the details), and we're not helpless to do anything about it, in either prevention or treatment.

Cancer is a disease of the cells, and what all of the more than one hundred known cancers have in common is wild cell proliferation that begins in a single mutated cell. That single cell evades the body's defenses and replicates unchecked. These new, proliferative cells—if unchecked (and the evidence indicates that they can yet be checked)—may eventually travel throughout the body, commandeer its organs, divert their energy supplies, and kill the "host"—us.

Carcinogenesis begins at the cellular level. All cancers apparently begin when the genetic material in a single cell becomes damaged by one or more of many different types of cancer-causing agents known as carcinogens. This mutated cell begins to multiply, eventually becoming the primary tumor.

As the primary tumor establishes itself—let's say in the liver—it also establishes an energy supply, creating new blood vessels that steal vital nourishment from the liver. This growth of new blood vessels to supply the tumor is one of the things that distinguishes a malignant, or cancerous, tumor from a benign tumor. (Benign tumors also result from mutant cells, but they are characterized by much slower growth that is usually self-limiting. For the most part, benign tumors do not take over the whole site or spread into surrounding tissues, although this is possible at a much slower rate.)

For a while, both the liver and cancer can coexist, but the growth of the mutated cells is so rapid that the tumor's hunger for energy soon outpaces that of the liver. Eventually, the liver is completely taken over—the tumor steals more and more of the energy supply and the liver can accomplish less and less until it is completely starved.

To get an idea of how a cancer works, imagine a pirate captain establishing a base of operations on an island. His pirate crew cuts down the native trees in order to construct the camp or burn them for fuel. They also steal food from the natives in order to feed themselves. The pirates enslave the natives and the natives begin to starve. Soon the pirates have taken over the whole island and quickly divert and absorb its energy supplies.

The process by which cancer spreads is known as *metastasis,* derived from the Greek meaning "to change states." Cells break off from the original tumor and spread through the bloodstream or the lymphatic system to different sites throughout the body. These metastatic cells are not just random cells that break off from the main tumor and float around until they happen to take hold somewhere. Indeed, the word *malignant* describes them all too perfectly: These colonizing cells are already adapted for growth at new body sites (perhaps by stealing genetic "maps" from the cells of the host organ), although the intricate genetics of this process aren't yet well understood. (Curiously, a cancerous cell that begins in, say, the lung, does not necessarily become lung cancer— it can migrate to another organ and take root there, becoming bladder cancer or liver cancer.)

Secondary tumors then do the same thing as the primary tumor: They establish themselves in the organ and divert and cut off its energy supply. This leads to a vast array of problems, including suppression of the immune system as normal metabolic function is damaged, leaving the victim susceptible to all kinds of infection, death of the organ (or necrosis), and internal bleeding. Any of these can kill.

To continue our analogy, the pirates realize that their energy supplies will not support them much longer. They get out their maps and set sail for other islands, to do exactly the same thing: colonize the island, commandeer its energy supplies, and set up a base for further operations. The pirates leave devastation in their wake: The unchecked growth of the primary tumor eventually destroys the host organ by completely diverting its energy supply. The same is true of secondary tumors.

If that description makes cancer sound inevitable and inevitably deadly, this is not so. Understanding what happens in the cancer process and when it happens is crucial to our being able to stop it before it starts. If cancer is a disease of the cells then it makes sense to talk first about cells and in general about how they work.

cells and cell division

We are cells, to coin a phrase, and cells are us. The entire structure of our bodies, from bone to skin, is cells, and our cells contain nearly everything we are—from the genetic code our bodies use to construct themselves to the microscopic power plants that burn the energy we consume.

At the very moment of conception, each of us begins life as a single cell formed from the union of egg and sperm (known as germ cells). This single, undifferentiated cell—the zygote—contains within it all of our genetic information. It goes on to multiply rapidly and transform itself exponentially into very highly differentiated and specialized cells that make up our various organs and tissues—bone, blood, hair, heart, fingers, liver, kidneys, and so on. In no time at all we transform: zygote, embryo, fetus, infant, child, adolescent, adult.

In many ways, understanding the growing embryo is instructive in understanding the cancer process, because while cancer is a disease of the cells, it is also a disease of energy (see chapter 6). In the nineteenth century, German physiologist Johannes Müller noted that the cells in cancerous tumors appeared to be quite different from normal cells. He found that they were much more similar to those found in developing embryos—they were characterized by rapid proliferation and a vast hunger for energy.

Once an embryo implants itself into the wall of its mother's womb, it establishes an energy supply, the placenta. The placenta grows along with the embryo. This is nature's plan. The placenta gets whatever nourishment the developing child gets from what is at large in the mother's bloodstream, and so it feeds not only off the mother's energy supply (what she eats) but off the mother's stores of energy and nutrients.[2] If the mother's diet is low

---

[2] Our bodies are constantly breaking down and rebuilding, which is why we can, through exercise and good nutrition, build stronger muscles and bones, and also why, through lack of exercise and good nutrition, build stores of fat, weaken our bones, and so on. Once our bodies have broken down our foods, the amino acids (the building blocks of protein) in our bloodstream, for example, become part of the same pool as amino acids broken down from muscle tissue.

in, say, calcium, the fetus will still get calcium from what is at large in the mother's body.

Like the embryo, one of the first things a cancer does, once it has evaded the body's natural defense mechanisms and implanted itself into the host organ, is to establish an energy supply. But while a fetus's growth may be rapid and hungry like the cancer cell's, its growth is programmed. In one sense, a cancer cell's growth is also planned, but it has no program to halt its growth. Indeed, a cancer cell's plan couldn't be more simple: grow and keep on growing. If you think of a cell as a car, it's built with both accelerator and brakes. Both a baby's and the mother's body know when it's time to put on the brakes—the baby is born. Built into our genetic code is the information to ensure that cell replication continues as it's supposed to continue, and stops when it's supposed to stop. A cancerous, mutated cell has an accelerator but no brakes. Once it has fuel and no obstacles, it will continue to put the figurative pedal to the metal and go. As we will discuss at length later on, for a mutated cell to get to this late stage, known as *progression,* requires a long and sometimes complex process.

That our cells know when and where to grow is one of the simplest (and most remarkable) things we can deduce from observing the growth of an embryo into a fully formed infant. For us to live, our cells must replicate. But as cancer is a disease of cell replication, clearly built into our survival are also the seeds of our potential destruction. Oncogenes, or literally "cancer genes," happen when a cell replicates and the genetic material that would act as the cell's brakes is mutated and fails. Rapid embryonic growth and hunger can ensue.

Even after we are fully grown the process of cell replication continues, except in certain long-lived proteins, which include the bones, muscles, and nervous system. Those organs and tissues that regularly interact with the environment are those where cancer most often takes place because these must replace or replenish themselves constantly: the skin, the lungs, the digestive tract, the kidneys and liver, the pancreas, and the reproductive organs.

These parts of us must continually cycle in and out of readiness for pregnancy and so require constant rejuvenation. But there are also parts of us that need to remain intact for as long as possible—if, for example, our nervous system were constantly having to replicate and replace itself, it would interfere with nerve transmission (imagine nerve impulses backed up in traffic while the body makes repairs to the nervous superhighway—it would result in paralysis). We would likely not have any substantial memory.

Cell division and replication, then, are fundamental to life. Even bones retain the capacity for cell replication if broken. (Unfortunately, nerves retain only shreds of their ability to replicate.)

The adult human's estimated 10 trillion cells are all derived from that first cell, and although each cell is highly specialized, each contains the whole of our genetic material. Along with a constant supply of energy and nutrients, that genetic material allows our bodies to perform this continual maintenance.

Our cells contain many different kinds of genetic information, but where the cancer process is concerned the important kinds of information are those that relate to growth accelerators, brakes, and genetic self-repair. When that genetic material is damaged, trouble can follow.

Cancer occurs only in cells that are replicating—those tissues mentioned above that must constantly cycle in and out of readiness. This is why the cancers that occur in children and young adults—who are growing and thus have cells replicating everywhere—tend to be different from those that occur in adults.

But how does cancer happen? How does an otherwise normal cell turn cancerous?

how cancer happens and how our bodies thwart it

Although this entire book is about how cancer happens and how our bodies thwart it—and how we can help them thwart it—in this section we will discuss the causes of mutant cells. We will also show how the portion of our immune system that is devoted to preventing mutants from continuing works. Researchers have not yet mapped out this process in its entirety, and much of it involves complicated molecular biology, so the material presented here is of necessity simplified and somewhat generalized.

Still, we can talk quite sensibly about what causes a mutation that could eventually lead to cancer.

The laboratory model of how a cell turns into a rogue mutant and becomes a tumor consists of three essential but overlapping phases: initiation, promotion, and progression. But while it is relatively simple to expose tissue in the lab to particular carcinogens, and then sit back and watch the cancer grow, the natural process of cancer is not as simple as one cell being hit by a carcinogen, going bad, and then proliferating into a tumorous mass.

In the real world—in our own tissues—these phases are more blurred and each has many potential variables. The first two phases can take decades to happen and can be affected for better or worse by many factors.

initiation

Initiation occurs when the cell is exposed to a carcinogenic compound, usually in steps and over many years. Again, the initiation process is not as simple as it sounds. There are many factors at work.

the attackers

There are many different ways that carcinogenesis can begin. Below are some of the things that can attack cells and cause mutation that leads to carcinogenesis.

- Inherited genetic traits (rare).
- Viruses and bacteria (human papilloma virus and *Helicobacter pylori* are examples).
- Attacking agents, or what we most commonly think of as carcinogens. These are chemical or cosmic forces, such as many of the chemicals found in tobacco smoke, and cosmic rays, such as ionizing and ultraviolet radiation.
- Over- or under-expression of growth-controlling genetic factors resulting from chromosome breakage. Growth-controlling genetic factors are those that govern the rate and extent of growth of our bodily structures. For example, our genes are programmed so that every organ grows "just so" and no more. When nutritional excess or deficiency causes loss or excess of certain chemicals, this can result in breakage of the DNA strand and a failure of the governing mechanism.
- Endogenous reactive compounds. *Endogenous* refers to chemicals that are produced within the body, and these would include oxides and nitrites created in the normal process of metabolism. (*Exogenous* refers to chemicals external to the body, and would include things like the compounds in tobacco smoke.)

the attackers' helpers

◆ Poor nutrition—dietary surplus or deficiency.
◆ Positive energy balance, e.g., obesity.
◆ Physical inactivity.
◆ Overabundance of hormones and other growth factors.

oxidation and antioxidants

Antioxidants, virtually unheard of ten or so years ago, have captured the imagination of researchers and the general public as a health necessity. But although nearly everyone has heard of antioxidants—and the market for supplemental antioxidants grows daily—few outside the health care industry or the research lab have a clear idea of what antioxidants are, what they do, or why they're necessary. Even researchers don't agree on how much of them we should have.

As you know, the metabolic process transforms energy through the use of oxygen into forms our bodies can utilize. A by-product of this transformation is oxidation, or the creation of molecules of "reactive" oxygen—oxides. As is true of many biological processes, oxidation is a good thing with the potential to become a bad thing. These oxides are unstable compounds, and up to a certain point their instability is a quality we actually use to our advantage. Think of those detergent commercials where the detergent "attaches" to dirt and "lifts stains right out." In the constant process of detoxifying our bodies, this is exactly how oxides work: They attach to waste products and destabilize them, leaving them in a state in which our bodies—assuming good, balanced nutrition and good overall health—can expel them. Far too many of us, however, do not get balanced nutrition. And when we eat too much in the way of energy foods and don't back them up with plentiful nutrient foods, the trouble with oxides arises.

Oxides are not "smart"—call them promiscuous. They'll attach to anything they can—and after a certain point, if there are too many of them, their instability can work to turn bodily compounds into toxic compounds. Indeed, reactive oxygen has the potential to damage the body by doing to it what it does to potentially harmful compounds: denaturing proteins, damaging nucleic acids in DNA, or saturating the double bonds of fatty acids in cell membranes, and basically turning our cells rancid. Any of these effects can increase cancer risk.

The potential for oxidation can be elevated by infections, vigorous physical activity (or overdoing exercise), or even excessive exposure to sunlight (UV radiation). The importance of antioxidants is that they ensure there are not too many of these reactive oxygen compounds roaming around the body.

To give an example of how an oxide can work to detoxify the body, take that staple of most medicine cabinets, hydrogen peroxide. This wonderful preparation helps to rid wounds of bacteria and can even be valuable in preventing tooth decay. You may know that every molecule has an electrical charge—it's this electrical energy that glues the molecules together, and this is the process by which magnetism works. Hydrogen peroxide, like any other oxide, is an unstable compound—that is, because of a free, or "open," electron, it's constantly trying to find another electron—like a magnet "looking" for metal to stick to. It's this property that makes it both valuable and dangerous. Bacteria tend to be stable compounds, and hydrogen peroxide mates with them and renders them unstable. When there are compounds like bacteria at large in the body, an oxide radical acts like those detergent bits attaching to particles of dirt, effectively neutralizing them—that's what all that fizzing with hydrogen peroxide is all about. Rendered unstable, the bacteria can be rinsed away.

If your dentist has ever recommended using peroxide as an oral rinse, it is for the same reason: It does a great job at destabilizing the bacteria that cause tooth decay so that they can be rinsed away. But your dentist probably also recommended that you take care not to swallow it. If you do, any oxides that have not been quenched or had their free electrons mated, will, once inside your body, continue looking to get quenched, because a free electron is a lonely electron.

This is a free radical. Countless numbers of these are created regularly in the metabolic process, as well as by exposure to environmental agents such as cigarette smoke and pollution, certain elements in food and drink, and sunlight. This puts the body under constant pressure to deal with them. This is known as oxidative stress, and this is why we need antioxidants. Although there are many, the two most important are vitamin C (water soluble) and vitamin E (fat soluble).

These unstable radicals will roam around the body as they were in part meant to, seeking out stable compounds to attach to and destabilize. This is good for the body so long as the compounds to which they attach themselves are waste products that need destabilization so they can be escorted out of the body, but not important players in metabolism or cell replication.

Aside from free radicals, there is another kind of highly energized, unstable "oxygen species" that isn't technically a free radical, because rather than a single electron it has paired electrons. It is also unstable and can destabilize other compounds. These include what is known as the "superoxide radical."

Fortunately, since our bodies expect certain levels of these compounds, they have developed considerable mechanisms (most of which are related to good nutrition and plenty of vegetables and fruits) to dispel these radicals and their spawn as necessary. Because our defense mechanisms are dependent upon a substantial, varied, and constant supply of antioxidants, poor or mediocre nutrition (even that which falls within the Recommended Daily Allowances) can allow these radicals free range in the body and cause considerable damage, DNA being a favored target.

As a matter of fact, oxidative damage to DNA occurs regularly, on a daily and even hourly basis. Most but not all of the damage is effectively corrected by our internal surveillance and repair systems. DNA is equipped with the means to render such damage meaningless—built into the genetic code is a backup blueprint for replicating the DNA without the damage. If the newly replicated DNA doesn't match the blueprint, the body eliminates it. But when damage occurs while DNA is replicating or during other vulnerable moments, and that internal blueprint is also damaged, this opens up the potential for mutations. It is then up to other surveillance and repair systems to fix that damage.

Other kinds of damage accrue in the oxidation of lipids that make up cell membranes. This damage to the cell membranes can eventually lead to DNA damage.

To get an idea of how diet, lifestyle, and nutrition come into this equation, think again of the example of detergent and laundry. Think of a white shirt or blouse you're fond of and wear frequently. Wear it gently (no changing the oil in the car), wash it gently and regularly, and it will have a long life. If you wear it constantly, and expose it to lots of things (like motor oil) that can stain or damage it, the only way you're going to get it clean is to use industrial-strength detergents, which may get it clean again, but the chances are the heavy-duty detergent will also damage the fabric and it will wear out sooner.

The same is true of the body and its own cleaning mechanisms. Overload it with free radicals from overexposure to the sun, fatty or highly processed foods, and allow it to become fat and lazy, and there will be an excess of radicals as the body works overtime to try to clean itself out. The radicals may be successfully eliminated, but they can also cause collateral damage from just those effects mentioned above.

They key is balance. You must do the equivalent of wearing your body gently: Exercise regularly; don't overeat; avoid pollutants, tobacco smoke, and other causes of unwarranted oxidative stress; and make sure your body is supplied with plenty of antioxidants, which are most plentiful in vegetables and fruits. This way, the body can maintain its metabolic equilibrium.

the role of antioxidants in stopping cancer before it starts

Antioxidants are microconstituents of diet involved in DNA and cell maintenance and repair. They protect the body against oxidative stress, including the attack from carcinogens.

Each cell has its own defense system that includes various enzymes and requires antioxidants. Carotenoids (vitamin A compounds such as beta-carotene—see "Phytochemicals and Bioactive Compounds" in chapter 9) and vitamins C and E scavenge reactive oxygen and quench oxidative chain reactions, preventing genetic damage in the cells. Antioxidants may also have nonantioxidant properties that protect against cancer.

the take-home message on antioxidants

Many bioactive compounds other than those mentioned above have antioxidant and other protective properties, but determining exactly which individual compounds in vegetables and fruits are responsible for decreasing cancer risk is not yet possible. Indeed, it may be the cooperation and interaction of many such compounds that decrease risk. This is why the take-home message on antioxidants has to be: Eat a constant and varied supply of vegetables and fruits. This will provide your body with the protective biochemicals it needs. This cooperation and interaction is also why it's important to get your antioxidants from the sources themselves and not from often-very-expensive supplements.

It's worthy of note that in addition to their role in cancer prevention, antioxidants have also been linked to prevention of cardiovascular disease and may well protect against diabetes mellitus, age-related eye diseases, degenerative nerve diseases such as Parkinson's, and possibly the aging process in general.

our built-in defenses

For the most part, carcinogens must be "initiated" in order to cause a genetic mutation, but even then they won't necessarily cause cancer. In general,
we have several layers of defense against cancer, just as we do against
other diseases. The first is genetic makeup, which, while we cannot change,
we can understand and minimize. Nutrition and lifestyle are the second
lines of defense, and they are the methods by which we can profoundly
affect any preordained genetic risk.

A dietary or lifestyle attacking agent is normally caught and escorted
out of the body by what are known as phase 1 enzymes. Phase 1 enzymes,
however, work in tandem with other metabolic systems (the albumin in the
blood system, for example, which works with the liver). Essentially, they
leave the waste products (including carcinogens) on the metabolic
doorstep to be picked up and carried off. To do this, they leave the compounds in a reactive state, which means they can react with DNA and
potentially cause damage to the genetic code. Phase 1 enzymes don't do
this to create mutagenic compounds; rather, they are making waste products more water-soluble and therefore more easily excreted. There are
many endogenous and dietary bioactive[3] compounds, particularly antioxidants, that will react with the activated carcinogens and render them harmless before they have a chance to react with DNA. Most of these are found
in vegetables and fruits, and if you don't eat them they won't be in your system to help out.

Some carcinogens are more potent than others. If a carcinogen
becomes activated, it is termed an *ultimate* carcinogen. By ultimate, it does
not mean that it is the supreme, all-powerful carcinogen, but that it has ultimately become capable of causing genetic damage.

The next line of defense, if a carcinogen becomes an ultimate carcinogen, are phase 2 detoxification enzymes. Phase 2 enzymes are turned on by
a variety of plant compounds (called bioactive phytochemicals). The more
vegetables you eat, the more your phase 2 enzymes will be active. Most

---

3 You'll see the term *bioactive* pop up again and again throughout this book. It simply indicates a
compound that has biological activity, which is a pretty vast category. While vitamins, minerals,
and other nutrients are all bioactive compounds, researchers are daily discovering increasing
numbers of constituents of foods that are bioactive but do not fall within such strictly defined categories. At some point in time, we will no doubt be able to categorize them more sensibly, but at
this point, the broad category must suffice.

often, the activated ultimate carcinogen is, again, escorted out of the body before it can do any damage.

If phase 2 enzymes are on a low state of alert, or are otherwise impaired and do not catch the ultimate carcinogen and send it packing, the compound can react with DNA and cause what are known as *adducts,* which can damage genetic material in three ways. First, they can distort the shape of the DNA, potentially causing mistranslations (imagine trying to make a tape recording of a record with a skip in it). Second, when the DNA replicates, the adducted base can be misread, causing a mutation in the new strand (a bit like that old game of Telephone or Gossip in which children sit in a circle and whisper something in the next child's ear). Third, repair of bulky adducts can cause breakages of the orderly DNA strand, which can in turn result in mutations or deletions of important genetic material (imagine a cat climbing your very delicate lace curtains).

The good news is there is yet another line of defense, and that is the DNA's internal repair mechanism. If you imagine genetic information as computer code, and mutagens as computer viruses (which are really much more like computer cancers), DNA has built into it an automatic backup and corruption detection. If information becomes corrupted, when the DNA "reads" information in order to replicate, it automatically spots and repairs any information that doesn't match the backup.

If this is so, why do we get cancer at all?

For one thing, this assumes that all systems are working at optimal capacity: Diet is supplying all the goodies your body needs to do these things, you're in energy balance (a concept we'll discuss), and so on. But if cells are reproducing rapidly, DNA can replicate before the repair is complete, passing onto the daughter cell the mutation. Mutations are therefore more likely to occur if DNA repair mechanisms are defective, as can be the case in inherited risk for cancer or if the repair mechanisms are impeded by a lack of the nutrients they need (many of which you won't find on any RDA charts) to work at full potential.

There are other kinds of repair mechanisms (many of which researchers are still working to puzzle out) for more extensive DNA damage, such as strand breakage and deletions, and failure of these mechanisms can also result in changes in the structure of the DNA.

When mutations or deletions happen in genetic material that is related to growth, growth suppression, and DNA repair, carcinogenesis can be the result.

Oncogenes can result when turned-off genetic growth material gets turned on again by genetic damage. Carcinogenesis can be the result. Tumor-suppressor genes are growth-controlling factors and part of the body's defense mechanism. If these become mutated and can no longer produce the appropriate protein, then carcinogenesis can result. The turning-off and turning-on of these important types of genetic material haven't been linked directly to any particular kind of dietary or nutritional factor. But it is entirely reasonable to assume that good, cancer-preventive nutrition, supplying plenty of the microgoodies that aid and abet good cellular function can work to prevent mutations.

Even when a cell turns mutant, there are still mechanisms by which the body can get rid of it. If DNA damage has occurred as a consequence of exposure to external carcinogens or oxygen radicals generated as a part of the metabolic process, and if the damage has persisted and has been passed on to a clone of daughter cells by cell replication, it is still possible for the damaged cells to die. All cells are equipped with a fail-safe cell-suicide mechanism (programmed cell death), which is intended to ensure the death of that cell if the DNA is damaged beyond repair. At some point in this accumulation of damage, the cell enters into the process known by the name of *apoptosis,* involving breakup of the DNA and death of the cell. It is distinguished from the cell death associated with tissue trauma (injury) or necrosis, by producing no inflammatory response.

It is now clear that the failure of some cancer cells to undergo apoptosis is the consequence either of loss of function of the tumor-suppressor gene and other genes that control the cell-cycle checkpoints, or loss of the integrity of the machinery of the apoptotic (cell-suicide) process itself.

Currently, there is no evidence to suggest that particular dietary or nutritional factors are related directly to how efficiently DNA repairs itself, but there is more than likely an indirect relationship. If your metabolism is running at peak efficiency through good diet, exercise, and overall health, then it's likely that various body systems, including DNA repair, are running efficiently as well.

In at least one type of cancer, a connection between diet and the apoptotic process has been noted. Recent laboratory studies suggest that volatile short-chain fatty acids (produced in the colon by the fermentation of fiber and complex carbohydrates) may induce apoptosis in colon cancer cell lines. Fiber and volatile fatty acids (or the lack thereof) are thought to be important factors in colon carcinogenesis, so the knowledge that proper fiber and its metabolic by-products can help stop cancer before it starts is important because it may help reveal other late-acting dietary modifiers of cancer in this and other organs. (Late-acting would refer to the relatively late portion of the metabolic process in which the creation of these fatty acids occurs.)

Whether or not you have a family history of cancer or some other known risk factor, the best defense is a good offense. In this case it's clearly best not to allow a carcinogen to get past the phase 2 enzymes. The most effective way of doing this is through diet, nutrition, and lifestyle choices that work with our defense mechanisms rather than against them. Eating vegetables is just a part of it. Energy balance and physical activity also play important roles. We will discuss diet, lifestyle, energy balance, and physical activity thoroughly in succeeding chapters.

promotion

The next stage in the cancer process is known as promotion. This occurs once a cell has been initiated. In this phase, certain chemicals or biological conditions that have no appreciable cancer-causing activity on their own can greatly enhance or promote the formation of tumors when they are consumed or when they occur in the presence of an initiated cell. Where carcinogens act directly, causing genetic mutations, tumor promoters appear to act indirectly, not so much by altering genetic material but by exerting an especially potent ability to cause cellular replication and profound changes in gene expression that alter controls on cell growth. In effect, they act a bit like co-conspirators, not exactly committing the crime of cancer but aiding and abetting it. They're the gas for the getaway car, the ammunition for the guns—or traitors who help the pirates gain a foothold on the island.

Once a cell is initiated, if it finds a favorable environment for growth—which would include plenty of energy and weakened defenses—then that single cell can be promoted into a definable tumorous mass.

In many respects, this middle phase of the cancer process is a crucial intersection of cancer with lifestyle and nutritional choices. This is because what we eat, how we eat, and how *much* we eat, as well as how much physical activity we get, all appear to affect how well our bodies will stop initiated cells before they become cancers—or whether they will at all.

chemical promoters

There are several different kinds of substances that act as promoters, some dietary, some environmental, and some endogenous, or produced by the body in the course of metabolism. Some of the chemicals that have been shown to act as tumor-promoters are (and you won't be quizzed on this): the phorbol ester derivatives (these are naturally occurring plant chemicals widely used in animal experiments that do not, for the most part, occur in conventional plant foods); certain barbiturate drugs (phenobarbital); chlorinated hydrocarbons from industry or agriculture (such as pesticides and industrial chemicals); and alcohol. Many of the noncarcinogenic chemicals in tobacco smoke also seem to have tumor-promoting properties, as do certain kinds of pollution. Hormones that our own bodies produce, such as human growth hormone (HGH), insulin, estrogen, and testosterone, can also have promoting effects—these are tissue-building hormones, and they don't necessarily distinguish between wanted and unwanted tissue. But the availability of such hormones for promotional activity appears largely to correlate with our metabolic balance. If you're physically fit and your diet is balanced in terms of providing energy and nutrition, then your hormones will likely be busy doing the jobs they're supposed to do and won't be loitering in your body's dark alleyways and corners, ready to make trouble.

Carcinogens themselves also seem to have promoting effects, although the mechanism for how they work may differ from agent to agent. It may be simply that the constant bombardment of particular cells by carcinogens, while not directly causing mutations, so overburdens our protective mechanisms that a favorable environment for tumor growth is created.

Alcohol is an interesting example of both a carcinogen and a promoter. Although identified as a class 1 carcinogen,[4] the numbers of cancers directly linked to alcohol, when compared with those linked to, say, tobacco, are considerably lower. But if you combine chronic use of alcohol with cigarette smoking, you get a wild increase in the likelihood of cancer over what might result from either by itself. (This is probably due to several things: the wide-ranging chemical effects of ethyl alcohol itself, the statistical likelihood that smokers and drinkers will consume a suboptimal diet, and also

---

4 Alcohol has been classified since 1988 by the International Agency for Research on Cancer (IARC) as a class 1 carcinogen for cancers of the liver and much of the upper aerodigestive tract: mouth, pharynx, larynx, and esophagus. (A class 1 carcinogen is the top rating of how likely a substance is to be carcinogenic in humans.)

the concentrated energy that alcohol provides, which at 7 calories per gram is second only to fat in its energy density.)

Additionally, high or low levels of essential dietary nutrients have themselves been shown to exhibit tumor-promoting activity. For example, experiments in which rodents were fed high dietary levels of protein, fats, or just plain old high-calorie diets from across the food groups, have shown classic tumor promotion activity as a result of positive energy balance. So over eating can help turn initiated cells into full-blown tumors. Not only does overeating provide lots of energy for cancers to grow on, but it overburdens metabolism in general. Obesity also throws off the balance of growth promoting hormones, mainly insulin, but also HGH and the others that interact with insulin as well.

The flip side of overconsumption is that nutritional deficiencies can also promote tumors. Moderate deficiencies of certain amino acids (the building blocks of protein) have been shown to enhance liver tumor formation in rodents quite significantly. For example, low levels of the essential amino acids methionine or choline have also shown classic tumor-promoting activity.

lifestyle

In addition to chemical promoters, there are also lifestyle patterns that have been shown to promote tumors. Lifestyle factors that can either enhance or inhibit promotion—even in a case where a cancer is linked to a genetic predisposition—are many. Studies that experimentally induce tumors in animals show that an increased intake of fat or calories in general markedly enhances the promotion of tumors in most tissues examined. Obesity and chronic energy surplus, mentioned above, are key, but lack of physical activity can also play a significant role.

If your body is running at peak performance, and your nutrition—particularly your intake of vegetables and fruits—is optimal, then you will put a minimum amount of stress on your immune system and its cancer-fighting elements. If you're constantly overeating, you're constantly loading up your body with potential toxins it must deal with, including oxides. In some respects, nearly everything you eat can have some toxic capacity—you can't have metabolism without having waste products of metabolism. Ideally what you do is minimize your body's load of toxins and maximize its ability to get rid of them. Overeating and underexertion both undermine this in several different ways. One is the ensuing imbalance of hormones mentioned above. Another is the indirect increase in oxidative stress (overloading your body with oxides and overwhelming its antioxidant defenses) and lipid peroxidation (turning the fats in your body rancid, including the lipoproteins that make up the membranes of your cells), which can lead not only to DNA damage and its consequences but also to a favorable environment in which tumors can grow.

genetic factors in promotion

It has become apparent that the different classes of *proto-oncogenes,* the growth-promoting genes that can become oncogenes when damaged, and the tumor-suppressor genes represent a network of genetic material that exerts intricate controls over growth processes. As this cellular machinery becomes damaged by exposure to carcinogens, radiation, and other tumor promoters, the potential that tumors will proliferate is increased.

To belabor our image of pirates just a bit more, imagine the proto-oncogenes as the island's potential traitors and the tumor-suppressor genes as the island's security force. If the pirates succeed in turning the potential traitors, the traitors can allow the pirates in. But if the security forces can exert enough influence, the traitors won't turn. If however, the security force is attacked and weakened by progressive assaults from the pirates, or if the security forces are disabled (by getting drunk or eating tainted food), the traitors may overwhelm them. If, when the pirates gain a foothold, the security force fails to rout them, then the pirates will have a better chance of taking over the island.

DNA's ability to repair damage in tumor suppressors or proto-oncogenes—or even in the genes that create the DNA-repair proteins themselves—will also affect the overall likelihood of any one cell turning mutant, and determine how favorable the environment is for promotion.

Other internal mechanisms that can act as promoters may include the proteins produced by the BRCA1 gene, the so-called breast cancer gene. This particular family of proteins is known to undergo changes that allow them to produce bioactive chemicals that will stimulate cell growth. These do not, however, fall into the same classes of genes that tumor suppressors and oncogenes fall into.

It is now apparent that each stage of carcinogenesis may be advanced further by carcinogen-induced DNA damage, as well as by certain conditions known as epigenetic mechanisms, that can alter the behavior of DNA without necessarily mutating it. As an example, viral proteins (such as those produced by the human papilloma virus) can bind to human cellular proteins that are produced by tumor-suppressor genes in a way that can allow uncontrolled growth even in the absence of a genetic mutation. Also, certain nutritional deficiencies can cause changes in gene expression in abnormal cells, resulting in the loss of control over growth. (Expression is sort of the genetic equivalent of a volume knob—a gene can be silent, or quiet, or it can scream, depending on the degree of expression.)

Although the picture of how genetics and promotion intertwine is far from complete, and much research needs to be done, we do know that diet and nutrition can profoundly affect how well genes behave themselves.

how our bodies work to defeat promotion

Just as certain deficiencies and surpluses can promote tumor growth, so can certain nutrients and lifestyle circumstances, in the proper balance, work to defeat tumor promotion.

NUTRIENTS

The beneficial or adverse effects of dietary components on tumor promotion and progression are frequently accompanied by decreased or increased levels, respectively, of oxidative damage in tissues that are potential cancer sites.

Studies have shown that a variety of different nutrients can be effective in delaying the progression of potentially cancerous lesions from one stage to the next. This is true of those in such disparate organs as the liver (by adequate but not overconsumption of the essential amino acids methionine and choline) and urinary tract (plentiful consumption of retinoids). Experiments have shown that retinoids[5] can, in cancers of the upper aerodigestive tract,[6] reduce the likelihood of a recurrence (or a second primary tumor) in people who have already been successfully treated for such cancers.

Some of the other nutrients that have shown protective effects against tumor promotion are selenium and vitamin D. This does not, however, mean that you should go out and buy supplements of these nutrients and

---

[5] These are vitamin A compounds. See "The Carotenoids" section of chapter 9.
[6] For example, the mouth, oropharynx, larynx, esophagus.

start popping them regularly. See the sections on vitamins and minerals in chapter 9.

Considerable speculation has centered on the possible role of oxidative damage to DNA in tumor promotion and progression, the natural damage that can occur as our bodies utilize energy. Evidence has accumulated associating DNA damage with increased energy intake.

The role of too much or too little energy (calories) has been seen to affect cancer in many studies. Energy restriction, or limiting the number of calories in the diet, has been shown in some laboratory studies with rats to suppress the formation of some tumors. Evidence of obesity's role in human cancers has been found in studies of breast, endometrium, colon, and kidney tumors. Physical activity, which maintains lean body mass as well as influences several other systems in the body, especially endocrine (hormone) and immunological function, is very consistently associated with a lower risk of colon cancer, and probably breast cancer. And given that cancer is a disease of energy as well as cells, it's likely that energy balance will affect most cancers.

Cell walls are constructed of proteins and fats, or lipoproteins, and the reactive waste oxides discussed previously can attach to fats—lipids—rendering them reactive as well. More recent studies have provided evidence that this can also eventually lead to DNA damage. It is now apparent that each stage of carcinogenesis may be advanced further by carcinogen-induced DNA damage, as well as by a variety of mechanisms that influence the behavior but not the structure of DNA.

progression

The last stage of the cancer process, progression, involves the increased growth and expansion of a population of initiated and promoted cancer cells from a focal lesion to an invasive tumor mass (the pirates taking over the island, with malignant behavior in mind), often accompanied by an increasingly abnormal complement of genetic material. DNA damage is widespread in this late stage, with loss, breakage, and duplication of multiple chromosomes. Progression leads ultimately to metastasis, whereby tumor cells migrate to distant sites in the body.

The role of food and nutrition, including carcinogens, in this final stage of tumorigenesis is not yet clear. Recent studies show that many chemical carcinogens and tumor promoters can give rise to the formation of reactive oxygen species that can cause DNA damage and chromosomal breakage; this is one mechanism that has been linked to the development of a fully malignant cancer. Agents that induce the early mutations may also contribute to the later stages of total disorganization of the tumor cell genome and the loss of control of proliferation and apoptosis. Although evidence for dietary agents that act in this way is lacking so far, epidemiological data on smoking suggest that tobacco-associated carcinogens could act both early and late in the cancer process.

By the time progression occurs, cancer has started. Our goal is to stop it before it gets this far. As noted, the best place to nip it is long before it has the chance to bud. And the best way to do it is by creating a healthier you.

3

some cancers and their relation to diet and nutrition

While it is impossible to say, "Eat food X and you won't get breast cancer," there is an undeniable relationship between diets high in, for example, vegetables and fruits, and a decrease in certain cancers. There is also a relationship between diets high in fats and sugars and a higher rate of certain cancers. Some of these links are known. Some are proven conclusively; others show evidence, but conclusive proof is not yet available.

Below is a list of some of the cancers most related to diet, lifestyle, and nutrition, and their known relationships to certain nutritional and lifestyle factors. Smoking and use of smokeless tobacco is a cancer-causing factor across the board, so for the most part it's been left out for simplicity's sake. Stopping the use of tobacco will improve your health immediately.

The following cancers are ordered more or less from top to bottom as they occur throughout the body. There is insufficient evidence to link all cancers to particular dietary or environmental causes, so only those cancers that have definable links are listed. Below each type of cancer is first listed known or suspected increasers of risk, and second, known or suspected decreasers of risk.

The list begins with cancers of the upper aerodigestive tract (mouth, pharynx, nasopharynx, larynx, and esophagus), then lung cancer, now the most common cancer in the world (an estimated 1.3 million people world-wide were diagnosed with lung cancer in 1996).

Following are cancers of the stomach, pancreas, and gallbladder. Pancreatic and gallbladder cancers are relatively uncommon but almost invariably deadly (although new operative techniques for pancreatic cancer, which is usually considered inoperable because of the delicate nature of the pancreas, are being developed).

Primary liver cancer comes next, followed by cancers of the colon and rectum, together the fourth most common cancer worldwide and of partic-ular concern in developed countries and urban areas of the developing world—and possibly the one most intimately related to diet.

Next are those that are sex-linked or hormone-related, including breast cancer, the most common cancer in women worldwide (although in this country lung cancer tops it), ovary, endometrium (the lining of the uterus), cervix, prostate (increasingly common in the developed world), and thy-roid (relatively uncommon).

Finally are cancers of the urinary tract, kidney, and bladder. The evi-dence of increased or decreased risk cannot be all-inclusive. Up or down risk factors are based on the best scientific evidence available. If there is no scientific evidence available at this point, this does not mean that it will not be available in the future.

For those factors that increase risk, reducing them when possible will help reduce risk. For example, if high intake of total fat is an increasing fac-tor, reducing the total fat in your diet would reduce your cancer risk.

Mouth and Pharynx
- There is some inconclusive evidence that the chronic consumption of very hot beverages may increase risk.
- A diet high in vegetables and fruits has been shown convincingly to reduce risk, while foods high in vitamin C may also reduce risk.

Nasopharynx (uncommon)
- Epstein-Barr virus and Cantonese-style salted fish are known to increase risk.

Larynx
- Evidence that alcohol increases risk is convincing, particularly in combination with tobacco.

◆ Avoid alcohol and eat a diet high in vegetables and fruits.

Esophagus

◆ Alcohol consumption. There is the possibility that deficient, cereal-based diets, very hot drinks, and certain chemicals formed in preserved foods (smoked, salted, cured) increase risk.

◆ A diet high in vegetables and fruits has been shown to decrease risk, and foods high in carotenoids and vitamin C have shown the potential to decrease risk.

Lung

◆ It is possible that overall consumption of fat, but particularly saturated fat, animal fats, and cholesterol, increases risk. Alcohol consumption may also increase risk, particularly in tandem with tobacco use.

◆ A diet high in vegetables and fruits has been shown to decrease risk; a diet high in foods that contain carotenoids has been shown to decrease risk. Physical activity and foods high in vitamin C, vitamin E, and selenium may decrease risk.

Stomach

◆ It is likely that a diet high in salt increases risk. It is possible that refined starch and grilled or barbecued meats and fish increase risk. There is insufficient evidence to know if cured meats and the chemical by-products of curing and grilling increase risk.

◆ A diet high in vegetables and fruits has been shown to decrease risk. Refrigeration (allowing a year-round diet high in vegetables and fruits and reducing the need for preservation) indirectly reduces risk. A diet high in foods containing vitamin C likely decreases risk, and a diet high in allium vegetables (onions, garlic, etc.), whole grains, and green tea may decrease risk.

Pancreas

◆ High energy intake, cholesterol, and meat may increase risk. The evidence that sugar, eggs, cured and smoked meats, and fish may increase risk is as yet insufficient.

◆ It is likely that a diet high in vegetables and fruits will decrease risk, and a diet high in fiber and foods rich in vitamin C also decreases risk.

Gallbladder

◆ There is insufficient evidence for dietary factors that decrease risk of this uncommon cancer, although it may be that obesity, through increased occurrence of gallstones and through its overall systemic effects, increases risk.

Liver

◆ Alcohol abuse that results in cirrhosis is a direct cause of liver cancer; aflatoxin contamination (from certain moldy foods) is likely to increase risk. Infection with hepatitis B or C is a nondietary cause. Evidence that excess iron consumption increases risk is insufficient.

◆ A diet high in vegetables may decrease risk. Evidence that foods rich in selenium decrease risk is insufficient.

Colon, Rectum

◆ A diet high in red meat and the consumption of alcohol are likely to increase risk. High body mass (obesity), greater adult height, frequent eating, sugar, total fat as well as saturated and animal fats, processed meats, eggs, and heavily cooked meats may increase risk. Evidence that excess iron consumption increases risk is insufficient. Nondietary factors that increase risk are certain genetic traits and inflammatory bowel disease.

◆ Physical activity has been shown to decrease risk, as has a diet high in vegetables.

◆ It is possible that a diet high in fiber, unprocessed starchy foods, and foods rich in carotenoids will decrease risk. The evidence that foods rich in vitamins C, D, and E, folates, or the amino acid methionine, and that cereals and coffee decrease risk is as yet insufficient.

Breast

◆ Rapid growth and greater adult height increase risk. High body mass (obesity), adult weight gain, and alcohol consumption are likely to increase risk (evidence is becoming clearer that they do). Total fat, as well as saturated and animal fats and meat may increase risk.[7] Evidence that DDT and other industrial chemical residues increase risk is inconclusive.

◆ A diet high in vegetables and fruits likely decreases risk. Physical activity, a diet high in fiber, and foods rich in carotenoids may decrease risk. Evidence is as yet insufficient to show that foods rich in vitamin C, the isoflavone micronutrients (such as those found in

---

[7] Three case control studies have reported significantly reduced risks associated with high consumption of olive oil. This evidence is also consistent with research in experimental animals. A rich source of monounsaturated fatty acids, which appear to bear no direct relationship to breast cancer, olive oil contains antioxidants such as vitamin E that may or may not have a direct relationship to breast cancer. It may be that if any protective effect of olive oil exists, it is due to the replacement of other fats that could increase risk.

soy products), lignins (the only dietary fiber that's not carbohy-drate), and fish decrease risk. The evidence that coffee consumption has no relationship to breast cancer is convincing. Having borne chil-dren decreases risk.

Ovary

◈ Evidence that total fat, particularly saturated/animal fats, and eggs increase risk is as yet insufficient. Low parity (having few or no chil-dren) and certain genetic abnormalities are nondietary factors known to increase risk.

◈ A diet high in vegetables and fruits will likely decrease risk. There is as yet insufficient evidence to show that a diet high in fish and carotenoids decreases risk. Having borne children is a nondietary factor that decreases risk.

Endometrium

◈ High body mass (obesity) increases risk. Saturated animal fats may increase risk. The evidence is as yet insufficient that total fat and cholesterol increase risk.

◈ Established nondietary risk factors are low parity and prolonged exposure to endogenous estrogens and to exogenous (external) estrogens (commonly used in hormone replacement therapy), partic-ularly without using exogenous progestogens at the same time. A diet high in vegetables and fruits may decrease risk, but the evidence that a diet high in foods rich in carotenoids decreases risk is as yet insuf-ficient.

Cervix (The incidence of cervical cancer mortality has been reduced considerably in recent years by widespread screening programs.)

◈ There is as yet no evidence that particular diet-related factors increase risk. Known nondietary factors that increase risk are HPV, or the human papilloma viruses, smoking, and sexually transmitted viral infection.

◈ It is possible that a diet high in vegetables and fruits, carotenoids, and vitamins C and E reduce risk.

Prostate

◈ It is possible that total fat, saturated/animal fat, meat, and dairy products increase risk. The evidence that high overall energy intake increases risk is as yet insufficient.

◈ A diet high in vegetables may decrease risk.

Thyroid (uncommon)

◈ Exposure to ionizing radiation (X rays, radiation from nuclear waste, and so on) is an established risk factor. It is likely that a diet deficient in iron increases risk; it is also possible that a diet too rich in iron increases risk. Evidence that high body mass (obesity) increases risk is insufficient.

◈ It is possible that a diet high in vegetables and fruits decreases risk. Evidence that a diet that is rich in selenium decreases risk is insufficient.

Kidney

◈ It is likely that high body mass (obesity) increases risk, particularly in women. It is possible that a diet high in meat, milk, and other dairy products increases risk.

◈ It is possible that a diet high in vegetables and fruits decreases risk.

Bladder

◈ Certain kinds of industrial or workplace exposures have been established as factors that increase risk, as has infestation with *Schistosoma haematobium*. It is also possible that consumption of more than five cups of coffee a day increases risk. Evidence that total fat, chlorinated hydrocarbons (most often found in industrial and agricultural chemicals and their residues), and fried foods increase risk is insufficient.

◈ It is likely that a diet rich in vegetables and fruits decreases risk. Evidence that a diet rich in foods containing vitamin C and retinol (vitamin A) decreases risk is insufficient.

nondietary risk factors for breast cancer

A number of risk factors for breast cancer have been established, most of which relate to "reproductive events," a category that includes not only birth but also miscarriage, the age of menarche, and not giving birth. Risk is increased by an early onset of menarche, nulliparity (not having children), late age at first birth, and late natural menopause.

To be precise, a longer reproductive lifetime that includes later and fewer (or no) births results in an increase in breast cancer rates. Although the exact mechanisms are not entirely known, the statistics implicate endogenous (internal) hormones, particularly estrogen, as the root of breast cancer incidence.

A family history of breast cancer is associated with about a twofold overall increase in incidence but there is a greater increase in risk if more than one close relative is affected, or if breast cancer has occurred at a young age in a family member. Inherited mutations of the genes BRCA1, BRCA2 and ATM have been identified by genetic researchers, and these convey a very high risk of breast cancer for the relatively small number of women affected. However, these appear to account for perhaps only 5 percent of all breast malignancies, which makes them accountable for only a very small portion of cancers overall.

Ionizing radiation (X rays, exposure to radioactive material, and so on) increases the risk of breast cancer, particularly when exposure occurs before age forty; this is probably a minor contribution to overall rates of breast cancer.

part II

creating a more cancer-resistant you

4

where are you on
the cancer prevention spectrum?

No, you can't cancer-proof yourself—not yet, anyway—but you can improve your health to maximize your chances of avoiding cancer.

When we speak of cancer prevention, we are not talking about early detection of cancer, nor are we talking about living a healthier life *with* cancer: We are talking about *stopping cancer before it starts*.

The information presented here is drawn primarily from the report *Food, Nutrition and the Prevention of Cancer: A Global Perspective*, the international study on diet and cancer produced by the American Institute for Cancer Research and its international affiliate, the World Cancer Research Fund. While that report was targeted at scientists and those involved in public health policy, the message it delivered is applicable to us all—*cancer can be prevented*.

The international panel that created that report reviewed thousands of the leading studies in the field of diet, nutrition, and cancer. They found overwhelming scientific evidence that cancer prevention is a very attainable goal, both for societies as a whole and for each of us as individuals.

The information that follows takes that report's findings and translates them into practical terms that can be used by you to make lower cancer risk a very real part of your life.

In this and ensuing chapters, we will show you how to take what you've learned so far about the mechanisms of cancer and apply that knowledge to your life to make yourself, beginning right now, more cancer-resistant. We'll provide you with ways of looking at where you are now and how you can begin to analyze your health balance so that—we hope—cancer doesn't happen to you at all.

Cancer prevention is a balance, ranging from the absolutely ideal (and probably impractical) to the high risk. Even at the ideal end of the scale, you won't be cancer-proof, but your statistical risk will be lowered considerably. Somewhere in the middle will lie the compromises that most of us have to make, because—let's face it—most of the time lifestyle is a balance between what we want to do and what we *have* to do.

Now that you know how cancer starts, and some of the ways nutrition and lifestyle affect it, let's take a look at your nutrition and lifestyle.

where are you now?

The nutrition and lifestyle adjustments you'll want to make to nudge yourself toward the ideal end of the cancer prevention spectrum will depend first on where you are now, and second on how far you're willing to go.

Where are you right now? What will you feel comfortable with? What can work in your life?

You may find that making small, incremental adjustments over time is much easier than trying to go from couch potato to triathlete tomorrow. Or, you may feel that the only way you can make changes is drastically. Perhaps, if you're already quite active, you might find that you don't really need to make too many changes to get yourself toward the ideal end of the scale.

Following is a list of several questions that will give you an idea if your cancer risk is different from that of the average population. When we talk about "average population," we're pretty much always talking about a mythical beast. What is average? If half the population is seven feet tall and half is five feet tall, then the average height of the population is six feet—

even though there's no one individual who's six feet tall. This does not mean, however, that *average* is useless. Far from it. As different as we all are, we all have things in common, and both the things we have in common and those we don't can provide us with a great deal of useful information, not to mention countless saved lives.

The point is, everybody differs slightly from the average—you know your body, you know your lifestyle, and you may therefore be the best judge of what's best for you.

When you answer these questions, it's important to remember two things:

First, risk is calculated based on statistics and probability—the law of averages. Second, cancer is many different diseases with many different factors that modulate it, and unless you've been snacking on plutonium, cancer—as you know from chapter 2—is rarely a foregone conclusion.

- Do you have a known genetically linked cancer in your family (for example, breast, ovarian, or colon)?
- If you're a woman, did you have your first period before the age of twelve?
- If you're a mother, did you bear your first child after age thirty?
- If you're a woman who's passed through menopause, are you on synthetic hormone replacement therapy?
- Did you gain more than eleven pounds after you reached full growth (about eighteen years old for women and twenty-four years old for men) and never lose it?
- Are you a woman over fifty who has never had children?
- Do you have inflammatory bowel disease?
- Have you ever been diagnosed with human papilloma virus (HPV)?
- Have you ever been treated for alcoholism?
- Have you ever been diagnosed with hepatitis virus B or C (HBV/HCV)?

If you answered yes to any of these questions, you may have a somewhat higher-than-average risk for certain cancers. You may already be aware of this and may have discussed it with your physician. What you may not be aware of is that even with a somewhat higher-than-average risk, there are steps you can take to help reduce your likelihood of getting cancer. With the largest number of cancers, *there is still something you can do.* Despite an increased statistical risk, *cancer is not inevitable.* Even the most dedicated smokers can reduce their risk of cancer simply by stopping.

If you answered yes to any of these questions and you are not already aware of an increased cancer risk, talk with your physician. You and your doctor may want to increase surveillance for any particular cancer for which you may be at somewhat increased risk—regular mammography, for example, or regular colonoscopy. But because your physician is probably not a nutritionist, read on: The guidelines in this book are of special value to you.

lifestyle or healthstyle?

When we talk about lifestyle in this country, we tend to think in broad strokes: "She's a tree-hugging vegetarian....He's a permanent bachelor slob....She's a soccer mom....He's a computer geek." These kinds of descriptions can be useful—if we're deciding whether or not to go on a blind date. But when it comes to analyzing lifestyle for ways we can improve cancer resistance, they're not much help.

The reality is, each of us is individually much more complex than any of these generalizations. You could easily be a tree-hugging vegetarian soccer mom who lives like a permanent bachelor slob and also happens to be a computer geek. But that still doesn't say much about you and cancer prevention.

Lifestyle—at least as it pertains to cancer prevention—isn't political affiliation, taste in music, or hairstyle. Lifestyle is something acquired over time, a cumulative force. It is, in a nutshell, the sum of everything we do.

The things we incorporate into our individual lifestyles are often unconscious, guided by habits so ancient they seem like instinct.

We humans tend to be creatures of habit, but habit is far deeper than simple, distinct behaviors like thumb-sucking or nail-biting. Indeed, habit extends deep into our culture and through all of our subcultures. Many of the things we do "instinctively" are in fact learned behaviors. Think of what you eat for breakfast, how you like your coffee or tea (or even *that* you like coffee or tea), the kinds of foods you automatically reach for when you snack, the kinds of sports you like to play or watch—all of these things are learned. To get an idea how important culture is to our habits, think of foreign travel. While part of its pleasure may be sight-seeing, more significant may be the immersion in a language and style of life that seem completely alien to our own—of being in a place, as the best-selling novelist John Irving once noted, where the mayonnaise comes in tubes. After travel, home never quite looks the same, because travel gives us the chance to stand outside ourselves and see more clearly who we are. If you can stand outside your lifestyle choices and look at them objectively, you'll have taken the first step toward being a more cancer-resistant you.

A more cancer-resistant lifestyle should probably be called a "health-style," because it is an educated one, with choices evaluated not only for convenience or pleasure or love or money, but also with the long-term goal of good overall health in mind.

Our behaviors, the things we do, follow patterns that we can each trace and understand. Start off with the species: There are certain things we do simply because we're human. Then follow with gender, culture, family, taste, education: All of our behaviors have influences and spring from these various wells. And so, if there are particular behaviors we would like to change, we can analyze the influences behind them and try to channel those energies in other directions.

The things that become part of healthstyle will be conscious choices guided by curiosity and research. We may, for example, use the stair-climber machine at the gym because we happen to know it will strengthen our leg muscles, help increase our ratio of lean body mass to fat, and improve cardiovascular as well as overall fitness.

If you're overweight or obese, there are probably a number of factors that have accumulated over the years to put you where you are today. Do you eat for reasons other than hunger? Do you snack daily on high-sugar, high-fat foods? Were both of your parents proto–couch potatoes? Do you sit and watch television during your spare time? Do you eat high-fat microwaveable frozen dinners for lunch almost every day? Does eating make you feel better when you're stressed out? Do you avoid physical exer-tion and feel hungry all the time?

All of these are learned behaviors, none of which alone is necessarily "bad." It is the accumulation of them—the pattern—that causes problems. They can be a vicious cycle. But you don't accumulate a lifestyle in a day, and you can't necessarily wave a magic wand and turn it into a healthstyle tomorrow. What you can do is address one or two at a time and gradually turn the cycle from vicious to virtuous.

By making changes a little at a time, over the course of a year or two it will seem like you did indeed wave a magic wand.

It is also undeniable that there are lifestyle elements that may have been forced upon us by circumstance. These we may not be able to change—nor, in many cases, will they be things that we want to change. For example, having kids creates certain realities and responsibilities we can't avoid, and most parents don't want to avoid them. Having a chronic illness, injury, or disability creates certain realities we must live with. But none of these means we necessarily have to live with a high risk of cancer.

evaluating your nutritional choices

Our primary biological reason for eating is nourishment—keeping the cells operating. But fueling up a human being is seldom so simple as pulling up to the pump, filling the tank, and pulling out (though in our time-crunched, hurried lifestyles it often may seem that way). We may select gasoline for its price, octane, etc., but it's not the way we usually select our foods. Our lifestyles influence heavily the things we eat and how often we eat them, as well as whether we burn the energy we consume or store it as fat.

Most of us have favorite foods, but most often they're our favorites not because of their perfect ratio of macro- to micronutrients (macronutrients are the basic nutritional elements, carbohydrate, protein, and fat; micronutrients are the vast array of vitamins, minerals, and other bioactive chemicals[8] we eat).

Favorite foods are likely associated with culture, family, and that infinitely complex and variable factor of personal taste ("I love sardines...I can't stand even the smell of fish"), as well as equally complex factors of emotional associations ("My mom used to make this for me when I was sick"). We also have considerable attitudes about foods, most of them based in family and culture.

If your parents came of age during the Depression and/or Second World War, they probably passed on many notions shaped by those years. From them you may have acquired notions about frugality—not wasting food,

---

[8] Again, in talking about "bioactive chemicals," we are mostly talking about chemicals that don't fall into conventional nutritional categories but are still important constituents of a cancer-healthy diet.

awareness that others in the world may be starving—or, if they wanted you to have everything they did not, you may carry precisely the opposite notions.

Whatever the case, keep in mind that attitudes about food and dietary patterns are learned and as such can be changed.

Chances are you eat many of the same sorts of foods your family ate when you were growing up, but chances are also good that you prepare them differently—you probably use less butter and fat; if you fry foods, you probably use monounsaturated fats such as olive oil or canola oil instead of shortening or lard. If you've made these kinds of improvements to the traditional family foods, you've probably done so because you know they are better for your health. But you, like many Americans, may harbor considerable confusion about what is good for you and what is not. We'll try to set you straight as we go. And you can refer to the recipes in the back of the book and start new family traditions today.

the nutrition unquiz

Many people are so accustomed to their lifestyle patterns that these patterns no longer even register. When talking to our doctors, we often misreport our food consumption because it's so unconscious. In some cases—gluttony being sinful—this may be deliberate. But often most of us just don't notice how much cream and sugar we put in our coffee, or how many doughnuts or sticks of chewing gum or bags of chips we grabbed on the fly during the last month. To take a closer look at your nutritional balance, start by looking at what you eat. Answer the following yes-or-no questions.

The natural thing to do when confronted with a list of questions like this is to view them as a test that must be passed. We tend to look for what the answers *should* be and answer accordingly. This is not a quiz. You can't pass or fail and the only one making any judgments will be you. There are no right or wrong answers.

1. Do you drink alcohol regularly (one or more glasses of wine, beer, or spirits on a daily or almost daily basis)?
2. When you eat meat, do you eat red meat more often than turkey, skinless chicken breast, or extra-lean meats?

3. When you eat red meat, is your serving size usually greater than four ounces?

4. Do you eat fish infrequently (less often than once a week)?

5. Do you skip breakfast almost every day?

6. Do you eat smoked or charcoal-grilled foods two or more times weekly?

7. Do you usually salt your food before even tasting it?

8. Do you eat salty foods daily or almost daily (including nuts, pretzels, chips, or salt-preserved foods)?

9. Do you include your snacks as part of your overall daily calorie and nutritional plan (for example, two of my snacks are two of my vegetable or fruit servings)?

10. Do you usually eat three to five servings of vegetables a day?

11. Do you usually eat two to three servings of fruit (not including bananas) or fruit juice a day?

If you answered yes to questions 1 through 8 and no to questions 9 through 11, your nutritional patterns may put you on the riskier end of the cancer-resistance scale, and you may find that you want to make some changes. But chances are pretty good that most people won't answer yes to all of 1 through 8 and no to all of 9 through 11.

Remember that while nutritional patterns are important to your cancer health by themselves, exercise can often go a long way towards offsetting less-than-ideal nutritional choices. But while you may keep your energy in balance, if you don't eat the all-important vegetables and fruits we'll discuss in chapter 9, you simply won't get the benefits of all the cancer-fighting microgoodies they supply.

In Part III, you'll get the complete skinny on the kinds of foods that are ideal and that you should be eating as regularly as possible, as well as those that are not so ideal and should be limited in every diet.

smoking

In any discussion of cancer resistance, it makes sense to talk about that single most cancer-unhealthy lifestyle choice: smoking. If you don't smoke and don't live with a smoker, skip ahead.

If you smoke, or use smokeless tobacco, stopping *now*—no matter how long you've been a tobacco user—will almost immediately improve your cancer risk as well as your overall health. In 1997 alone, the American Cancer Society estimates that nearly 175,000 people died from tobacco-related cancers. Other estimates put the overall number of tobacco-related deaths as high as nearly half a million.

If you *want* to get cancer or heart disease, damage your immune system, and pretty much thoroughly poison yourself, there is almost no single better way to do so than smoking. Although smoking is most often associated with lung cancer—a very real danger—numerous studies have linked smoking to many other cancers, including cancers of what is known as the upper aerodigestive tract, or the various pipes and valves that make up the connection between our lungs and stomach to the outside world: mouth, tongue, nose, throat, esophagus, larynx, epiglottis, etc.

Studies have also shown that cancer risk for smokers is increased significantly if the smoker drinks alcohol, even in small amounts.

Nicotine is a strange and powerful drug. It seems to act as both stimulant and depressant, and smokers apparently learn unconsciously to use it in both ways by inhaling differently, depending upon mood. Mood alteration is why nicotine is addictive, and for many people, nicotine seems to make it much easier to control moods and mood swings. In fact, there was a significant push in the last several years to end smoking in all public institutions, but researchers found that in the case of mental hospitals, ending smoking by patients frequently worsened their mental condition. In certain cases of individuals with severe depression, some researchers now recommend that these smokers not stop—nicotine is such a powerful mood regulator. In a sense, these smokers have discovered the power of nicotine as a mood regulator and have been self-medicating in order to stave off the disorder. But severe depression is relatively rare and there are newer, much safer medications that can help. If you find yourself depressed when you try to stop smoking cold turkey, talk to your physician about other, safer methods of mood regulation—these can range from prescription medications to relaxation and meditation techniques.

If you try to stop and have a relapse, don't worry, try again—many people who stop successfully fail at least once or twice before succeeding. Indeed, this failure may be an integral part of the stopping and not failure at all.

If you only smoke "socially," or when you're out with friends, you're still a smoker, at least as far as cancer risk goes. When you smoke, you're drawing some four thousand *identified* compounds into the deepest recesses of your lungs. The same is true if you're forced to be a passive smoker. As far as cancer risk is concerned, the best thing you can do is keep smoke out of your lungs.

Remember, smoking is an addiction, and addiction is not just chemical dependency: It is a three-part problem that involves psychological factors (self-medication), lifestyle factors (the circumstances under which you smoke), as well as physical dependence on the drug. When you kick the habit, you are significantly altering all of these things.

If you've tried to stop cold turkey and cannot, nicotine-replacement therapy (using nicotine gum or patches) has been shown to increase the likelihood of success significantly. If you've tried nicotine replacement therapy and haven't had much success, talk to your physician about other methods available. The FDA has recently approved a nicotine nasal spray that has been very effective in clinical trials, and there are also other prescription, nonnicotine methods currently becoming available. The newest at this writing is Welbutrin, shown to be more than twice as effective as stopping cold turkey, but has the added benefit of not being addictive. Still, it's a rule of thumb with prescription and even over-the-counter medications that nearly any given drug can have side effects.

Consider also joining a twelve-step or other addiction-eliminating program, which can be found through the American Cancer Society (1-800-ACS-2345) or often your local hospital. While alcoholics have long found the support and companionship of Alcoholics Anonymous to be invaluable in stopping drinking, most smokers stop alone. However, studies have shown a much higher success rate among those who have emotional and moral support from others like themselves. (It's worth mentioning that the same is true of people who are trying to lose weight.)

how cancer-protective is your current lifestyle?

Although some of us may have an above-average risk of cancer because of factors we cannot change, recent studies show that most of us (even those of us with recognized risk factors, such as the BRCA1 gene) can be as cancer resistant as we want to be—or can be within the limits of our lifestyle. (We should hasten to point out that this doesn't mean that if you get cancer, it's your fault. Being able to manipulate variables doesn't mean being able to *control* them.)

Does your current lifestyle predispose you to a greater risk for cancer, or does it serve to protect you? Like nutritional choices, lifestyle choices tend to be matters of habit. Many of them may be of necessity as well, dictated by job or family or even disability.

What sort of job do you have? Does it require you to be on the road (or in the air) a lot? When you're on the road, do your normal nutritional and fitness patterns go out the window—do you find yourself grabbing a bite, whatever happens to be convenient, rather than having a meal you've planned? Do you leave your jogging clothes behind or do you use the hotel weight room or pool? Do your family and work responsibilities leave you feeling so time-crunched that you can't get a moment to exercise? For recreation, do you prefer indoor activities such as building models, doing needlepoint, or watching television over outdoor activities such as gardening, walking, fishing, bird-watching, or kite-flying?

As with nutritional choices, our lifestyle choices are learned behaviors influenced by family, culture, and taste. We often don't so much need to unlearn them—if that's even possible—as we need to *re*learn them, reshape them, get *them* into shape.

It's not likely that a single week without exercise or a weekend of really delicious, high-calorie desserts is going to give you cancer. It's the accumulation of no exercise over time, of high-calorie desserts on a regular basis, and so on that will increase your risk. Would it be more ideal if you didn't let a week go by without exercising? Yes, provided you're not ill. And would it be more ideal if you never touched another really delicious, high-calorie dessert? Yes. But these things are not likely to give you cancer, either.

Think of it this way: If you use your health as a bank account, all the healthful things you do will accumulate and pay off dividends now and in the future, helping to prevent cancer and chronic disease, slow down aging, avoid or recover quickly from infectious illness, and so on. If you never make deposits, your account will be empty. If you use your health as a charge account, borrowing against good health by neglecting nutrition and exercise, doing foolish things like smoking and bingeing on alcohol, becoming overweight or obese, then down the road you may have to face the finance charges of clogged arteries, carcinogenesis, and so on.

the lifestyle unquiz

Following is another list of yes-or-no questions. Again, this is not a quiz and there are no right or wrong answers. Answer these questions as honestly as you can.

1. Do you smoke or use smokeless tobacco products?
2. Are you above your ideal weight[9] for your size and build?
3. Have you allowed chronic illness (diabetes, arthritis, etc.) to limit your physical activity?
4. Does your job require you to sit in a chair eight hours a day?
5. Are you too time-crunched to exercise?
6. Do you work up a sweat at least three times a week?
7. When time-crunched, do you make time for exercise anyway?
8. Do you walk short distances instead of drive?
9. Do you take the stairs instead of the elevator or escalator for three or fewer flights of stairs?
10. Can you spring up a flight of stairs without getting winded?

If you answered no to questions 1 through 5 and yes to questions 6 through 10, you may just possibly be perfect. If you answered 1 through 5 yes and 6 through 10 no, you may seriously want to consider making some changes in your lifestyle. But chances are, if you're like the average American, you had a no or two where a yes would have been healthier, and vice versa.

If you smoke, stop. If you're not sure if you're overweight, or aren't happy with the way you look in a bathing suit, see "The Body Mass Index" that follows, and chapter 6.

If you're too time-crunched to exercise, you may not really have a good handle on your lifestyle, or you may have some common attitudes or misconceptions about exercise that you can change. (See chapter 5.) Try to be aware of your physical activity as you go through your day: Are there places and ways you can work in more physical exertion? There are probably more than you might think.

---

[9] Ideal weight, like many averages, is a mythical beast. Ideal weight according to the actuarial charts for a man at a particular height may be 175 pounds. If a man of that height is a serious athlete, he may weigh considerably more—muscle is a lot heavier and denser than fat. An athlete's bones are also more likely to be denser. So in some sense, you will have to determine what your own ideal weight is based on your lifestyle, body mass, and other very subjective means. See pages 71 and 72.

how does your body measure up for cancer prevention?

We humans are notoriously terrible at self-awareness. This may result from self-consciousness and timidity, believing we are less than we are; or from hubris and arrogance, believing ourselves to be a lot more perfect than we are. The old adage has it that women look in the mirror and see nothing but imperfection; men look in the mirror and so long as they can suck in their gut they see nothing but perfection.

In the following pages, we will offer a few different ways of giving yourself a more objective (but still necessarily subjective) view of how you measure up. Remember, however, that everybody is different, and while one person could be 5 feet 5 inches tall and weigh 130 pounds, he or she could have a considerably different percentage of body fat than someone of the exact same height and weight. If you used only one index, you may be misclassified if you're exceptionally fit, or exceptionally sedentary, or smoke, and so on. So by using two or three measures, you can get a more three-dimensional picture of how you measure up.

If you smoke, you can pretty much throw everything out the window. Stop, and then give yourself a couple of months (you'll probably gain some weight, but you'll also probably lose it later) and then come back and measure yourself.

While being an ideal weight has its importance, what's really important in your physical makeup is the relationship between lean body mass (muscle is dense and weighs more, inch for inch) and adipose tissue (or fat, which is pretty flabby and takes up more space).

It's important to have some body fat—it is not only a store of energy, it also serves a lot of protective functions such as cushioning organs, helping you stay hydrated, and so on. But it's also important to have a good ratio of lean body mass to fat in order to keep all your systems in balance and running at optimum levels.

Speaking very generally, the higher your percentage of lean body mass, the healthier you're going to be overall—although having no fat at all would not be good. Recommendations for average people are that women carry roughly 20 to 25 percent body fat and men 15 to 18 percent.

Even if you're skinny, you may not have a very good ratio of fat to lean body mass, particularly if you smoke, drink regularly, or rarely exercise. Whether you're shaped like an apple, a pear, a potato, or a banana, where you are now will give you a clearer picture of where you can go.

the body mass index

Body mass sounds a little like a term borrowed from astronomy—perhaps a mathematical formula for calculating planetary movement. But when we say, "What's your body mass?," we're really saying, "Are you the right weight for your size?"

The ideal way to measure your body fat percentage would be to undergo a lot of expensive tests—floatation studies (fat floats better than muscle), bone density analysis, and so on. But even in epidemiological studies, these aren't very practical. Unless you're a professional athlete, or a movie star with a personal trainer and access to a lot of technology, it isn't very likely that you'll get such an exacting measurement. The good news is that it isn't necessary.

The body mass index provides us with a means to figure out roughly how big we are as opposed to approximately how big we ought to be. Bigness, in this sense, is the relationship between height and weight. The more you weigh at any given height, the higher your body mass. The body mass index provides a formula for figuring your own body mass index (BMI) and is the measure most commonly in use these days (although the MetLife charts still have considerable value).

The body mass index uses metric measures, so we've provided a table in feet and inches so you don't have to calculate the formula yourself. If you want to, it will give you a slightly more exact index, but you'll still want to use the other "tests" or measures.

In the following table, you'll find the body mass index along the top. Find your height. (Do any of us really know how tall we are? You can find an approximate height or look at those you believe are closest to your height if you don't actually take off your shoes and measure yourself.) Then find your weight (weight tends to vary throughout the day, depending upon your intake of food and drink, and your bowel habits). It's best to measure your weight at the same time every day (in the morning, for example, dressed but with no shoes). Follow the line from your height all the way over to your weight. Look at the top BMI numbers, and that's your body mass index.

The healthy range is considered to be a BMI of 18.5 to 25. A BMI of 30 or over is considered obese.

BMI	19	20	21	22	23	24	25	26	27	28	29	30	35	40
4'10"	91	96	100	105	110	115	119	124	129	134	138	143	167	191
4'11"	94	99	104	109	114	119	124	128	133	138	143	148	173	198
5'	97	102	107	112	118	123	128	133	138	143	148	153	179	204
5'1"	100	106	111	116	122	127	132	137	143	148	153	158	185	211
5'2"	104	109	115	120	126	131	136	142	147	153	158	164	191	218
5'3"	107	113	118	124	130	135	141	146	152	158	163	169	197	225
5'4"	110	116	122	128	134	140	145	151	157	163	169	174	204	232
5'5"	114	120	126	132	138	144	150	156	162	168	174	180	210	240
5'6"	118	124	130	136	142	148	155	161	167	173	179	186	216	247
5'7"	121	127	134	140	146	153	159	166	172	178	185	191	223	255
5'8"	125	131	138	144	151	158	164	171	177	184	190	197	230	262
5'9"	128	135	142	149	155	162	169	176	182	189	196	203	236	270
5'10"	132	139	146	153	160	167	174	181	188	195	202	207	243	278
5'11"	136	143	150	157	165	172	179	186	193	200	208	215	250	286
6'	140	147	154	162	169	177	184	191	199	206	213	221	258	294
6'1"	144	151	159	166	174	182	189	197	204	212	219	227	265	302
6'2"	148	155	163	171	179	186	194	202	210	218	225	233	272	311
6'3"	152	160	168	176	184	192	200	208	216	224	232	240	279	319
6'4"	156	164	172	180	189	197	205	213	221	230	238	246	287	328

height (in feet and inches)

weight (in pounds)

Reprinted with permission, Tufts University Health & Nutrition Letter, April 1997

If you want a more exacting measure than the table provides, this is how you do it:

Say you're 5 feet tall and your weight is 120 pounds.

- ◆ Multiply your weight in pounds by 700. Result: 84,000
- ◆ Square your height in inches. You're 60 inches, so your result is 3,600.
- ◆ Now divide the multiple of your weight by the square of your height (84,000÷3,600). Result: a BMI of 23.3.

If you exercise regularly, you probably have more muscle and denser bones, and so you will have a higher BMI. Don't worry about it—everybody is different. But if you're not an athlete and your BMI is still above the healthy range, you will probably need to adjust your energy balance.

the fruit index

Certain kinds of body fat (particularly that which is centered around the waist, known variously as visceral fat, abdominal adiposity, and android adiposity) are associated with higher risk not only for cancer but for heart disease, diabetes, and other potentially life-threatening chronic illness. So where your fat is located can be as important as how much of it you have.

The American Heart Association and American institute for Cancer Research recommend, among other measures, an estimation of abdominal fat by what kind of fruit your body shape resembles: are you an apple or a pear? Here's the "fruit formula" for coming up with your "fruit index":

1. With a tape measure, measure your waist. In this case, waist isn't necessarily where your belt buckles. (Men, trouser size doesn't equal waist circumference.) Use your navel as the start and finish point for your tape measure.
2. Now measure your hips at their widest point.
3. Now take the measure of your waist and divide it by the measure of your hips. You can do this with a pocket calculator and you should come up with a small number. For men, the number, or your fruit index, should be less than one—that is, you're an apple, or approaching applehood, if your waist measure is equal to or greater than your hip measure. For women, your hips are naturally bigger than your waist, so your ideal fruit index is going to be less than 0.8—0.8 or greater means that unless you're naturally small-hipped, you're an apple. If your index is lower, you're a pear.

Having an apple versus a pear shape (your waist to hip ratio) does give you a good idea of whether you have the type of adiposity (a nice way of saying flab) that is associated with increased risk of all sorts of illness, including diabetes, cancer, heart disease, and stroke. Having a high fruit index (an apple shape) means you probably need to lose weight. But even if you're shaped like an artichoke, your shape doesn't tell you the entire story about how much weight you need to lose—or if indeed you need to lose weight. It just gives you an idea—which you may already have had.

the metlife tables

Figuring out where you are in the weight balance is where the MetLife tables come in handy. The tables will give you a roughly appropriate weight for your frame. The versions of the tables here are those published in 1959 and not those revised and published in 1983 (which were revised because heavier people were living longer). The American Heart Association and other health groups still use the older tables because even though people may be living longer, excess body weight is still a health problem and cause of disease. We include the older tables here for the same reason—because our concern is disease prevention. Cancer risk has been linked to body fat (and the kinds of foods and lifestyles that produce it) again and again. Interestingly, it was in the 1930s that some of the first rock-solid statistical evidence that diet and cancer are related came to be known. Insurance companies, collecting actuarial data on their customers, found that those who were overweight consistently had higher rates of cancer and other chronic diseases.

using the metlife tables: are you large, medium, or small framed?

The first step is to figure out what your frame type is—are you of large, medium, or small build? You'll need a ruler for this test.

◆ First, extend your right arm in front of you, palm up.

◆ Now bend that arm at the elbow so that arm and forearm form a right angle.

◆ Using the thumb of your left hand, locate the bone on the inside of your elbow.

◆ Now, using your hand like a caliper, place the forefinger of your left hand on the bone that pokes out at the corner of your elbow.

◆ Keeping your left hand frozen in this measurement, remove your right arm from your left hand, pick up the ruler, and measure the distance between thumb and forefinger.

◆ In order to gauge your frame type, use the table below. If your measurement is lower than the ranges listed, then you're small-framed. If it's higher, then you're large-framed. If it falls within the ranges, then you're medium-framed.

elbow measurements for medium frame

HEIGHT IN 1″ HEELS MEN	ELBOW BREADTH	HEIGHT IN 1″ HEELS WOMEN	ELBOW BREADTH
5'2"–5'3"	2½"–2⅞"	4'10"–4'11"	2¼"–2½"
5'4"–5'7"	2⅝"–2⅞"	5'0"–5'3"	2¼"–2½"
5'8"–5'11"	2¾"–3"	5'4"–5'7"	2⅜"–2⅝"
6'0"–6'3"	2¾"–3⅛"	5'8"–5'11"	2⅜"–2⅝"
6'4"	2⅞"–3¼"	6'0"	2½"–2¾"

Reprinted courtesy of Metropolitan Life Insurance Company, Statistical Bulletin

Now you should have a pretty good notion of where you are, but where do you go from here?

Are you over your ideal weight for your size? Is your body mass index high for your size? Are you an apple and not a pear?

Have you noticed, as you've read, some things about your lifestyle that you think probably need changing?

If you're right in a sensible weight for your frame, that's probably good. But even if you are the ideal weight, have an appropriate BMI, and are the "right" kind of fruit, there are likely few of us who do not have aspects of lifestyle and diet that we could change for the better. For example, statistics show that most of us don't come anywhere near the number of servings of vegetables we ought to have per day, and as we'll discuss in chapter 9, vegetables are the richest source we have of cancer-fighting nutrients. There's no evidence at all that you can overdose on vegetables, so no matter how many vegetables you eat you could probably work into your diet another serving or two of spinach or broccoli.

But if you're overweight, even slimming down a *little* can have considerable health benefits. So the next thing to do is take a look at physical activity.

height & weight table for men

HEIGHT	SMALL FRAME	MEDIUM FRAME	LARGE FRAME
5'2"	128–134	131–141	138–150
5'3"	130–136	133–143	140–153
5'4"	132–138	135–145	142–156
5'5"	134–140	137–148	144–160
5'6"	136–142	139–151	146–164
5'7"	138–145	142–154	149–168
5'8"	140–148	145–157	152–172
5'9"	142–151	148–160	155–176
5'10"	144–154	151–163	158–180
5'11"	146–157	154–166	161–184
6'0"	149–160	157–170	164–188
6'1"	152–164	160–174	168–192
6'2"	155–168	164–178	172–197
6'3"	158–172	167–182	176–202
6'4"	162–176	171–187	181–207

height & weight table for women

HEIGHT	SMALL FRAME	MEDIUM FRAME	LARGE FRAME
4'10"	102–111	109–121	118–131
4'11"	103–113	111–123	120–134
5'0"	104–115	113–126	122–137
5'1"	106–118	115–129	125–140
5'2"	108–121	118–132	128–143
5'3"	111–124	121–135	131–147
5'4"	114–127	124–138	134–151
5'5"	117–130	127–141	137–155
5'6"	120–133	130–144	140–159
5'7"	123–136	133–147	143–163
5'8"	126–139	136–150	146–167
5'9"	129–142	139–153	149–170
5'10"	132–145	142–156	152–173
5'11"	135–148	145–159	155–176
6'0"	138–151	148–162	158–179

Weights at ages 25-59 based on lowest mortality. Weight in pounds according to frame (indoor clothing weighing 5 lbs for men and 3 lbs for women; shoes with 1" heels)

Reprinted courtesy of Metropolitan Life Insurance Company, Statistical Bulletin

5

cancer and exercise:
exercise may not be what you think

Imagine a new miracle cure that would:

◆ help you lose weight, lower your blood pressure and your cholesterol, and improve your circulation.
◆ help you sleep more soundly, concentrate better at work, and lift
your depression.
◆ help you live longer and healthier by reducing your risk of cancer
and cardiovascular disease, obesity and diabetes, osteoporosis and
arthritis, as well as a host of other diseases.
◆ improve your sex life *and* your social life.

You don't need to imagine it because it's real, and you don't need to line up
for hours, mail by midnight tonight, or have your credit card handy,
because not only is it cheap—even free—it's available wherever you are,
whenever you want it.

Good old physical activity—exercise—can be nearly whatever you want it to be, as long as you *move*. And although many of us believe we don't have the time for exercise, the reality is that working physical activity into our days is easy, and can if necessary be had in bits and pieces. If we can make *as little as twenty minutes a day* for exercise, it's like money in the bank. And the benefits of exercise increase in proportion to its frequency and its strenuousness, so if you can devote as little as one hour in twenty-four to this "miracle cure," the benefits will accrue accordingly.

cancer and fitness

Pinpointing the exact effects of fitness on cancer risk is not easy because people who are physically fit tend to have healthier lifestyles overall. Several studies, however, suggest that physical activity itself is critical in cancer prevention. Exercise broadly affects metabolism, but its key role in helping to prevent cancer may be the role it plays in balancing the calorie equation. As we will discuss in the following chapter, cancer is a disease of energy, and opportunistically seems to spring up a lot more readily in obese and overweight bodies where energy is in plentiful supply.

the evidence so far

In several studies, scientists have observed that people who live sedentary lifestyles have a higher risk of developing colon cancer than their more active counterparts. Confirming these findings, a long-term study of college graduates coordinated by Stanford University scientist Ralph S. Paffenbarger, Jr., M.D., found that alumni who were moderately to highly active had about half the risk of colon cancer compared to those who were inactive. Dr. Paffenbarger reports that the exercise doesn't have to be all *that* vigorous. "You don't have to be a marathon runner. However, there is a need to be up on your feet, moving about and using the large muscles every day."

Rose Frisch, Ph.D., professor emerita of the Harvard School of Public Health, found that women who participated in college athletics had a 35 percent lower rate of cancer of the breast and a 60 percent lower rate of cancer of the reproductive system in later years than those who had not been involved in athletics. Why?

Again, it's not entirely clear, but Dr. Frisch believes that the female athletes in her study burned more calories and were leaner as a result. "Fat makes estrogen, so leaner people make less estrogen. They also make a less potent form of estrogen," she explains. That shift in estrogen production is critical, says Dr. Frisch, because some of the cancers that women develop depend on estrogen for growth.

Dr. Frisch points out that it's not pounds that seem to make the difference, but body fat (the all-important ratio of fat to lean body mass, or muscle). Two people who see the same number on the scales may have very different proportions of body fat to lean body mass—and therefore very different cancer risks. The distribution of body fat (the fruit index we discussed in the last chapter) may also have an impact: fat around the waist, for example, may pose a greater risk than fat on the thighs.

The results from animal experiments on exercise and cancer have been mixed. Several studies have found that exercise protects against breast and pancreatic cancer in animals. However, Dr. Henry J. Thompson, deputy director of the AMC Cancer Research Center, found that low level aerobic exercise actually increased the incidence of breast cancer in rats compared to rats that were not exercised. Does this mean women should avoid exercise? "My studies show that a certain level of exercise increased the development of breast cancer in laboratory animals. Yet other studies, using other exercise regimens, have shown a protective effect," answers Dr. Thompson. "Since exercise offers so many positive health benefits, a better question might be: Which type of exercise is most protective?"

The varied results of animal studies point not only to the need for additional research in which different types and degrees of exercise are examined, but also the differences between humans and research animals. Scientists are calling for more research in humans to determine the type, timing, frequency, intensity, and regularity of physical activity and its influence on cancer risk. Once researchers better understand the relationship between exercise and cancer in people, they may be able to quantify more readily what cancers are impacted by what specific types of physical activities. But despite any conflicting findings in animal research, it is clear that fit bodies develop fewer cancers, and physical activity and good nutrition are the cornerstones to fitness.

you don't need steel buns to be fit—or to lower cancer risk

Since the early 1980s, when the government recommended lowering our intake of fats because of the link between fats and chronic disease, Americans have indeed reduced their intake of fats—but we have not gotten slimmer. Despite the so-called fitness craze, as a nation, we've actually become fatter—the numbers of overweight and obese Americans have skyrocketed. But packing a spare tire is not exclusive to Americans. As noted in the previous chapter, both American and British insurance companies have increased "ideal" weights to reflect the increasing girth of their respective citizenries. If we are reducing fat intake, why has this happened?

There are likely many reasons. First is that while fat intake may have fallen, overall intake of calories has not. Over the last fifty years, the numbers of fast-food chains have skyrocketed, as has our intake of these very high calorie, low nutrition foods. Add to that the epidemic of "sedentarism" that has steadily crept up on us over the last few decades. Where once we simply could not avoid physical exertion, today physical activity, like so many other things, becomes the lifestyle choice of exercise—one that's all too easy to jettison. When the going gets hectic, the hectic get fat.

In addition, the character of work as we understand it has changed dramatically in the past fifty years. We employ indoor plumbing, electricity, and all sorts of wonderful machines that take much of the physical strain from our daily lives. It used to be that strenuous physical activity was simply a reality of nearly everyone's everyday life. As our economy has turned more toward an information and service-oriented model and as appliances have taken over many of the tasks that were once a reality of everyday life, the character of work, has changed dramatically.

The character of play has also changed dramatically. Who, a hundred years ago, could have imagined sitting motionless and staring at a piece of furniture for hours? Yet that's exactly what we do when we watch television. And research into children and TV has shown that the metabolic rate of a child staring at the tube is actually *lower* than that of the same child asleep! While certainly people used to entertain themselves in a more or less motionless position a hundred years ago—reading, listening to music—they also had less time to do it, and did other things such as dancing to amuse themselves.

To get an idea how work has changed, consider something as simple and everyday-ordinary as laundry, which today may be little more than background noise as we put clothing or linens into the machine, then move the load to the dryer when the cycle finishes. The only strenuous part is going up and down the stairs—if your washing machine happens to be in your basement.

In the past you would have had to heat tubs of water for washing and rinsing, agitate the soiled clothing by hand, rinse it, wring it (either by hand or by running it through a mechanical wringer), dispose of the dirty water, then hang the clothing out to dry. And then, of course, before the advent of permanent-press fabrics, everything had to be ironed.

A hundred or even fifty years ago, much of the work available was agricultural, manufacturing, or other types of manual labor that required regular physical exertion. Once it might have taken several men several days to excavate the foundation for a new house. Today a single person sitting in a bulldozer can do it in a matter of hours. Much of today's information and service professions, by contrast, tend to be mentally and emotionally stressful—getting a new software operating system up and running, dealing with finicky and often difficult customers, meeting deadlines, and so on. But these tasks are too often not physically strenuous.

For those of us who don't have desk jobs, automation and mechanization have rendered much of our work considerably less strenuous than it once might have been. Our bodies evolved over millennia to deal with all sorts of drudgery—we needed to consume large amounts of energy because we burned large amounts of energy. Today we have not adjusted our metabolic makeup at all to match these vast changes. But how do we deal with today's abundance of energy and the few opportunities to burn it? This freedom from drudgery should be cause for celebration. Today the variety of foods available to us year-round is unequalled in history; today the variety of physical activities is astonishing. Yet the number of Americans who get just twenty minutes a day or less of merely *moderate* exercise is remarkably low and growing lower. According to the Surgeon General, the number of Americans who report regular, sustained activity is less than 20 percent; the number who report engaging in regular vigorous activity is less than 15 percent. Those who report no activity at all is nearly 30 percent.

This may go hand in hand with the reality that statistically we are aging as a nation—and it's almost a rule of thumb that the older we get, the more responsibilities we have, the busier we are, and the less time we have for ourselves. Older, retired people who do have the time to invest in fitness may feel that they deserve a rest. While this may very well be true, resting should most certainly not mean becoming sedentary. Weight gain of more than about five to ten pounds in the later years is a marker not just for cancer but for chronic disease across the board. Most of us, unfortunately, can look at family albums and marvel at how slim we all used to look.

It is sad that a lot of us equate exercise with work, for this really should not be the case.

Research clearly shows that making fitness time for ourselves increases not only the quality of life by reducing stress, improving immune function, and so on, but also increases the *quantity* of life.

What's your outlook on fitness? After seeing countless gleaming, well-muscled models and athletes on TV working their steel buns off and saying foolish things like, "No pain, no gain," have you concluded that you could never possibly measure up? Or do you intend to exercise more but never quite get around to it? Or have you decided that you're not the fitness type, and that exercise only falls into a few strict categories available only to a fitness elite?

This misperception is as harmful as it is wrong. The chief difference between work and fun isn't the amount of exertion involved, but the level of pleasure. So if it helps you to move, don't think of exercise as a workout, think of it as a *funout*.

While some kinds of exercise/recreation/physical activity such as hiking or biking may in themselves be pleasing—being in the wilderness, watching the seasons change—there is also a distinct physical pleasure in the mere act of exertion. Indeed, our bodies provide built-in physical and emotional rewards (such as the well-documented runner's high) for using them. Ever spend a day skiing or hiking or kite-flying with the kids and fall into bed utterly exhausted, but also utterly high over your accomplishment? If nothing else, exercise can give you a concrete sense of accomplishment that many of us do not get anywhere else. Many professions and even many personal endeavors seldom offer the sense of reward that exercise does. In a day of pushing paper (or manipulating information), or even in a day of parenting, can you stand back and look, and say what you accomplished? Perhaps. But exercise gives you constant rewards. Whether it's running, lifting weights, mowing the lawn, walking with your mate, gardening, or skiing, you can look back at what you did with a sense of joy and pleasure.

is yours a sedentary lifestyle?

If you do lead a sedentary lifestyle, you probably never started out think-ing, *I want to be a couch potato when I grow up.* If you're like most of us, you were probably an active kid. Exercise of one variety or another was just part of your routine—running around with friends, jumping rope, walking to class from your dorm, going on biking or hiking outings, tossing a ball or Frisbee in the afternoons, going for long, conversational (not to mention romantic) walks with friends or your future mate.

And if you're like most of the sedentary population, a sedentary lifestyle just crept up on you slowly. Now you may be in the position of grabbing your leisure when you can get it—an hour or two in front of the TV, an evening with your church group or reading club, a night out for din-ner and a movie while a baby-sitter holds the fort. Exercise, or at least what you commonly think of as exercise, doesn't really make it into the picture.

You don't *have* to be sedentary, but neither do you have to have buns of steel to be fit—and to reduce your risk of cancer.

While the *ideal* goal is to be as physically fit as possible while being as close to an ideal weight for your body type, physical fitness only occasion-ally correlates one to one with an ideal physical appearance. Can you walk up two flights of stairs without breathing heavily, but still you carry a hint of a spare tire? Studies have shown that we mistake physical appearance for all sorts of things it's not—the point is, don't think you have to look like a dancer to dance, like a runner to run, like a gardener to garden, or like a swimmer to swim.

There is even a level of physical activity that's appropriate for those who are disabled, for those who suffer from chronic conditions such as arthritis or diabetes or even cardiovascular disease, or those who have just been sedentary for a long time.

And not only will physical activity improve your physical condition, it will improve your emotional outlook as well—indeed, exercise is often rec-ommended in the treatment of depression.

Remember, however, that whenever you begin an exercise program (especially if it's a temporary and potentially strenuous one such as raking leaves or shoveling snow) you should check with your doctor to find out what level of exertion is appropriate for you. If you've been sedentary for a while, you may need to take it slow when you start.

Before we talk about ways that you can work physical activity into your healthstyle, let's take a look at where you are now.

take a moment to assess your fitness

Where are you now when it comes to staying physically active? Do you drive when you could walk? Do you take the elevator when you could take the stairs? Do you sit for most of the day? When you come home from work do you drive to the grocery store? Carry your groceries in a pushcart, then drive up to the parcel pickup lane to load them? When you're home, does exercise consist mainly of going from the kitchen to the dining room to the family room and then to bed?

All of that—sitting in traffic, preparing meals, cleaning up after supper, worrying over bills, and so on—has the potential to be pretty exhausting; but it's mentally exhausting, not physically exhausting. So it's no surprise that many of us, when we need to unwind mentally, flop down in front of the TV, surf the Web, or curl up on the couch with a good book before bedtime. While these may provide some escape from stress, stress is a physiological reaction[10] and venting it is best done with physical activity.

What is your fitness level now? Are you exerting yourself sufficiently to maintain good health and lower your cancer risk? Or are you having trouble just getting off the couch?

The following test is like the ones you encountered earlier in the book. It's not going to be graded. No one but you will evaluate the results. If you're honest with yourself, you can get a better idea of what you can do to nudge yourself further into the cancer-protective side of the spectrum.[11]

---

[10] Stress as we know it is actually an accumulation of stress reactions, part of our bodies' "fight or flight" mechanism. In this mechanism, your body releases stress hormones, which in turn unleash energy. If you're angry at your boss or a customer, if you're confronting a new and strange situation, these days most often you're neither going to fight or flee. Most of us, unfortunately for our bodies, just suck in and accumulate those stress reactions. This constant accumulation can result in all of the symptoms of stress—sleeplessness, irritability, uncontrollable emotional outbursts, high blood pressure, and so on. And it can impair immune function and have all sorts of other unpleasant metabolic side effects. The single best way to relieve stress is not through medication but exercise. Meditation breathing exercises, and other such outlets can also be beneficial.

[11] This simple test was devised by the certified personal trainers and owners of Fitness That Works, Inc., in Chantilly, Virginia.

1. Which of the following best describes your activity level *during the past three to six months?*
   A. I participate in physical activity, such as brisk walking, jogging, swimming, cycling, weight lifting, and/or sports such as tennis, basketball, or handball, for a minimum of twenty minutes at least two to three times a week.
   B. I participate in modest physical activity, such as golf, horseback riding, calisthenics, table tennis, bowling, or yard work, at least two to three times a week.
   C. I do not regularly participate in recreational activities, sports, or other types of physical activity.

2. I make an attempt to increase my daily activity by taking the stairs instead of the elevator or parking my car a distance from the office or store:
   A. always. I get a little something in almost every day.
   B. occasionally—two to three times a week.
   C seldom or never.

3. I can walk at a relatively brisk pace (fast enough to tax my breathing, but not so fast I can't talk) without having to stop:
   A. for thirty minutes or more.
   B. for ten to twenty minutes.
   C. for 5 minutes or less.

4. When I walk up one flight of stairs:
   A. it doesn't bother me.
   B. I feel somewhat winded.
   C. I feel very winded and fatigued.

5. When I get up from a comfortable couch or easy chair:
   A. I have no problem.
   B. I have to maneuver a little to get up.
   C. I have difficulty getting up.

6. If my car is parked across the parking lot and I'm carrying two full bags of groceries:
   A. it might be a little difficult, but I wouldn't need to pull up the car.
   B. I could probably make it to the car, but my arms would hurt and I'd be out of breath.
   C. I would have to pull the car up because there's no way I could handle them alone.

7. I stretch my muscles or take a stretch or yoga class for at least fifteen minutes:
    A. regularly, three to six times a week.
    B. about twice a week.
    C. never.
8. I experience low back tightness:
    A. never.
    B. during the day.
    C. upon awakening.
9. I can balance on my dominant (stronger) leg for:
    A. fifteen seconds or more.
    B. between five and fifteen seconds.
    C. less than five seconds.
10. Overall, I feel good about myself, my lifestyle and eating habits, and my fitness level:
    A. always.
    B sometimes.
    C. never.

score yourself:

A = three points
B = two points
C = one point

  ◆ 25 to 30: Congratulations! You've been taking pretty good care of yourself. But then you probably already know that and that's why you feel as good as you do.
  ◆ 16 to 24: Not bad! You've been making some pretty healthy lifestyle choices. But it might be time to reevaluate how and where you get your exercise in order to increase the intensity or duration, or maybe even change the type of exercise you're doing.
  ◆ Below 15: Uh-oh. You're sedentary. You should take this as a wake-up call for better health through better fitness.

where do you go from here?

For nearly all of us, the only place to go is up, even if you are already quite active. To get an idea of where you need or may want to go from here—what "up" is—it's helpful to know your physical activity level. The test above should give you an idea of what your physical activity level is. The AICR/WCRF expert panel, in its report on cancer prevention, recommends that to maintain health and reduce cancer risk we each have a minimum physical activity level (or PAL) of at least 1.75 or more.

pal

What on earth, you may sensibly wonder, is a PAL, a physical activity level, of 1.75. If you scored 25 to 30 on the preceding fitness test, then you are probably enjoying a PAL of 1.75 or above. If you scored in the lower ranges, your PAL may occasionally reach 1.75, but is more likely in the 1.3 to 1.6 range.

PAL is a way researchers express how much energy an individual expends. As you know, just being alive takes a certain amount of energy.

Arriving at your PAL takes into account the amount of energy, or number of calories, your body burns to keep the cellular fireplaces at least smoldering—this is your "basal metabolic rate" (BMR)—and then adds to it a multiple of that amount of energy. So if you have a PAL of 1.75, then you're burning 75 percent more than your BMR. If you have a PAL of 2.0, then you're burning twice your BMR. If your PAL is 1.3, then you're burning only 30 percent more.

For the most part, this multiple, like all of the other exacting formulas you met in the last chapter, is a "guesstimate." While it is possible to figure these things exactly with lots of measurements and scientific equipment, for purposes of gauging your cancer-fitness, the guesstimates are just fine. The goal is not to analyze down to the last decimal point, but to give you an idea where you are and where you can go to improve your health and cancer-resistance.

Basal metabolic rate is in some ways a mythical beast: it includes nothing but a base amount of energy, and is a representation of how many calories a waking body will use and no more, not the energy it takes to get up and answer the door, climb into bed, turn on the TV, or run around the neighborhood. The only reason you need to figure your basal metabolic rate is in order to get an idea of what your PAL is and how you can increase it.

getting to pal

To get to your PAL, you can really guess, based on the test above, or you can use the fascinating equation known as the Harris-Benedict scale. In order to use this scale, you'll need the following information: whether you're a man or a woman, your weight in pounds, your height in inches, and your age in years. Simple.

The next thing to do is take this simple information and plug it into the simple but strange equation below. Just for the sake of demonstration, we're going to use a "PAL pal," or a fictional 45-year-old, 5-feet, 120-pound woman, to walk you through the steps not only of BMR but also PAL, just so you won't go NUTS.

Here's the Harris-Benedict equation. You can refer to it later if you like Below it is the translation into practical terms.

> *Women:*
> 655
> + 4.36 x weight in pounds
> + 4.32 x height in inches
> - 4.7 x age in years
> = BMR

> *Men:*
> 66
> + 6.22 x weight in pounds
> + 12.7 x height in inches
> - 6.8 x age in years
> = BMR

how you do it: bmr in practical terms

First, take your weight in pounds and, if you're a woman, multiply it by 4.36 (6.22 for men). So for our PAL pal gal, 120 x 4.36 = 523.2

Second, take your height in inches and multiply it by 4.32 (12.7 for men). So 60 x 4.32 = 259.2.

Third, take your age in years and multiply it by 4.7 (6.8 for men). So 45 x 4.7 = 211.5

Now, add 655 (66 for men—don't worry if the figures 655 and 66 seem vastly different, they're correct) to the first and second figure—655 + 523.2 + 259.2 (= 1437.4), and then subtract the third figure, 211.5, from that (1437.4 - 211.5 = 1225.9).

So, our 45-year-old PAL gal, who stands five feet tall and weighs 120 pounds, has a BMR of 1225.9. This is how many calories she needs to burn just to maintain her, shall we say, standard of living. As noted above, it is necessarily imprecise because everyone has a different metabolism, and perhaps the two most important aspects of metabolism are your ratio of fat to lean body mass and your level of fitness, both of which will likely go hand-in-hand. The higher your PAL, which we shall discuss in a moment, the higher your BMR is likely to be.[12]

One of the reasons it makes so much difference to your BMR whether you're a man or a woman is that men have a naturally higher ratio of lean body mass (muscle) to fat. This has to do mainly with hormonal balances. Testosterone, an anabolic or tissue-building hormone, is the chief tissue builder in both men and women. Men have more of it by nature than women. (Illegal anabolic steroids abused by foolish athletes to build muscle are usually variations on testosterone.) A body with a higher percentage of lean body mass naturally burns more calories than a flabby one, even though overweight people may breathe more heavily and their hearts may race on that trip to the refrigerator.

What happens in an overweight, sedentary body is roughly this: if you don't move around very much but eat a lot, in effect you put your body into a state hibernation. Your body will store energy and be very stingy in using it. This is one of the reasons why people who diet without exercising to lose weight often find it difficult to do so—their bodies get even stingier. The evolutionary history of our species is one of periodic famine and hardship, and so our bodies, expecting such conditions, want to salt away energy for

---

12 There are of course folks who really earn the title "fitness crazed" who figure out to the calorie what their BMR is by measuring everything they eat, measuring their own weight over a period of time, and measuring their activities, and so on, then doing the necessary math. As noted, you can do this too, if you want, but you don't need to.

when it's no longer so readily available. Then when it does become unavailable, our bodies are stingy about giving it up. No one's body is built with the metabolic expectation that this sort of hibernative state is going to last. These periods of plenty have the evolutionary history of being shorter in duration than periods of hardship. Today's western, industrial diet doesn't normally include periods of hardship and famine and can lead to the vicious cycle of fat-and-fatter. As we shall discuss in Chapter 6, this energy surplus has a profound impact on cancer health.

To get back to PAL and BMR, if you're very active, your BMR is actually likely to be higher—it takes more calories to maintain muscle. If you're sedentary, your basal metabolic rate is likely to burn fewer calories.

If you're part of the huge population segment who's sedentary, then your PAL is likely to be around 1.3 to 1.6. Let's say our PAL pal gal has a PAL of 1.5. That is, she burns 50 percent more than her basal metabolic rate of 1225.9 calories, or about 613 calories. This means that, if she is like most Americans today, she's likely going to be in a positive energy balance, or

average calories burned in 10 minutes (of continuous activity)[13]

ACTIVITY	BODY WEIGHT IN POUNDS/CALORIES BURNED		
	120-130	160-170	190-200
Aerobics	60-105	75-140	90-165
Bicycling			
• outdoor	40-145	50-195	60-230
• stationary	25-145	30-195	40-230
Dancing	30-80	40-105	45-120
Gardening	30-80	40-105	45-120
Jogging			
• 5 mph (12 min./mile)	90	115	135
• 6 mph (10 min./mile)	105	140	165
Swimming	50-125	65-165	75-200
Walking			
• 2 mph (30 min./mile)	30	40	45
• 4 mph (15 min./mile)	55	70	85

13 SOURCE: "Walk Your Way to Fitness," Supplement to Mayo Clinic Health Letter, 1992, with permission of Mayo Foundation for Medical Education and Research

consuming more calories than she's burning, a concept we shall explore thoroughly in the next chapter. To get up to 1.75, she's going to need to add sufficient activity to her lifestyle to burn an additional 307 calories a day. Opposite is a table of a variety of common activities with a range of average calories they will burn in ten minutes. From the numbers of calories each of them burns, you can extrapolate to other exercises that are roughly the equivalent. Canoeing, for example, might be roughly equivalent to cycling, while hiking would probably fall between walking and jogging.

Using the table, our PAL gal will want to add to her current schedule an average of about 310 calories worth of exercise per day. This might, depending upon her preferences, work out to 30-40 minutes of aerobics, or an equivalent amount of steady swimming, dancing, gardening, or other activities. She could shorten the duration of her activity by increasing the strenuousness of it. If she's too busy to work in specific blocks of exercise time, she can change elements of her lifestyle to get in equivalents: carrying her groceries to the car (or better, walking to the grocery and carrying the groceries home), walking up the stairs at the office, or using an exercise machine at home while reading or watching television.

turning your sedentary lifestyle into an active one

Just like our PAL gal, there are lots of ways you can increase the amount of physical activity you get without really changing your lifestyle (except the sedentary part of it) too much. If you start out by incorporating modest activity into your daily routine, such as walking, raking leaves, climbing up stairs, or taking ten-minute walking breaks (instead of coffee breaks), you can accumulate fitness. Or you can try recreational activities like golf, tennis, or bowling, then gradually increase their intensity or length.

If you've been sedentary for any significant period of time (6 months), or if you're over forty or have any kind of chronic condition, before you start any kind of fitness program, it's best to check with your physician to make sure that your program of choice is going to kill you. Your physician can help you decide what level is appropriate for your age, weight, and health.

It's also important to keep in mind that before doing any activity such as jogging, biking, swimming, or even walking, it makes a big difference if you stretch before and after. Proper stretching exercises can significantly reduce the likelihood of injury, and they will also improve your overall flexibility and reduce the likelihood of muscle and joint aches and pains. If you have no idea how to stretch, you can look in your local library for books on the activity you intend to pursue, you can join a health club and talk to their fitness trainers, and you can talk to your physician to see what she or he recommends. Many health care organizations offer lots of information on keeping fit, so if you belong to an HMO, talk to them and find out what sort of information they have available.

the take-home message on cancer and fitness

Nearly any kind of sustained, regular physical activity is good for you whether you sweat or not, but activities that make you sweat have been shown to provide more health benefits than those that don't. This doesn't mean, however, that you need to sweat rivers (always make sure you keep adequately hydrated). The recently-reported results of the Physicians Health Study, which has followed some 22,000 male physicians since the mid-1980s, found that the risk of heart attack fell some 36 percent in those who exercised vigorously for 11-24 minutes, twice per week. The risk fell even more among those who exercised more. Those who did so 5 or more times per week had nearly a 50 percent reduction in risk.

While this study followed only men, similar studies have shown similar benefits for women.

One of the most interesting aspects of the Physicians Health Study was that it showed that those who exercised regularly, even if for relatively short periods, had the most benefit. And while low-sweat or no-sweat activities are probably the ones that appeal to most of us, there are lots of reasons to consider more vigorous activity. For those of us who lead hectic lifestyles, perhaps the best news is that more vigorous activity requires less time to provide the same benefit.

A *New Yorker* magazine article explored the conundrum of the Arizona tribe of Native Americans known as the Pimas, who have been studied extensively by diet and health researchers because of their high levels of obesity, diabetes, and cardiovascular and other related disease. Some Arizona Pimas can weigh as much as 500 pounds. Their plight grows worse with each decade. While the intricacies of the Pima question are no doubt quite complex, one of the most prominent reasons for their high levels of obesity and illness is lack of exercise. A sister tribe, geographically separated from the Pimas hundreds of years ago but genetically quite similar, lives in the mountains of Mexico. These Pimas are anything but ill or obese. Quite slim, actually, they are subsistence farmers whose diet is much what it has been for centuries. But these Pimas actually consume on average, *more* calories per day than the Arizona Pimas. The chief difference between the two groups seems to be attitude (the Arizona Pimas, according to researchers, have one of hopelessness and the inevitability of their plight) and levels of physical activity.

The research is clear that those who exercise regularly have a lower incidence of cancer (and other disease) than those who don't. This does not mean that exercise will necessarily cancer-proof you, but it will make cancer less likely. If you do get cancer, good overall health is going to make recovering from cancer (or other disease) much easier.

So the choice is up to you: gardening, dancing, splitting wood, skiing, hiking, landscaping, swimming, walking, jumping rope, car washing, horseback riding, karate, housecleaning, ice-skating, going up and down stairs, walking to your car or the grocery, ditch digging, biking, sex[14]—the list can be nearly endless.

If you decide to spend the money and invest in a home gym or other home exercise equipment, you may want to join a health club or the "Y" for a period of time in order to find out whether you like to ride a stationary bike, use a stair-climber, or other equipment. There's little reason to sink five hundred to one thousand dollars or more into a machine you don't like to use. And check out buyer's guides to such equipment to see how different brands and models are rated and how they might meet your expectations.

A final note: One of the great contemporary marketing schemes is the so-called energy bar, intended for hikers and bikers and active people. This is often not much more than a candy bar disguised as healthy food, even those made from honey and whey protein and other healthy stuff. If you eat a balanced diet, there's very little likelihood that you'll need one of these unless you're doing a triathalon. In a one hour jog, you'll burn a maximum of about one thousand calories. If you have an energy bar, which can contain as many as fifteen thousand calories, before or after your jog, it's pretty easy to do the math and figure you'll end your healthful jog having consumed more than you've burned.

---

14 The idea that athletes make better lovers has considerable truth to it. If you have more stamina, more energy, better circulation, and feel better, feel better about yourself, you may feel like making love more often, and may well become a better lover.

6

cancer and energy

Energy, as noted earlier, plays a crucial role in the cancer initiation and promotion process. Without energy there is no growth and no cell replication—without energy there can also be no life. So the key to optimum health is what is known as energy balance.

what is energy balance?

For human beings, the negotiable currency of energy comes in the forms of glucose and triglycerides (sugar and fat). These we calculate in calories, which are a measure of heat. As we discussed in the previous chapter, each of us must burn a certain number of calories in order to maintain basal metabolic rate, or BMR—those necessary functions of respiration, circulation, digestion, and so on that keep us alive. And so that means we must burn (and thus have stored or consume), a minimum number of calories per day.

If calories, pure and simple, were all we needed—the way a car needs only gasoline—life and diet would indeed be easy. But even a car needs more than gasoline—otherwise there would be no such thing as mechanics. A car, just like our bodies, needs a certain level of preventative maintenance. Your mechanic will do this for your car, but who does it for your body? Your physician can help you do some of it, and you'll do some of it consciously (like brushing your teeth, exercising, and choosing your foods wisely). But most of it your body does on its own, provided you keep up your end of the bargain and supply it with the materials to do so. In this regard, physical activity and nutrition are the primary tools your body needs to keep up these functions.

Energy, like many things in life, needs to be in balance in order for bodily systems to work properly. Overfill your gas tank, put in too much oil, and you not only have a mess, you can seriously damage your car. However, the elegant process of metabolism is more complex than just fueling up and burning the fuel. The word *metabolism* itself derives from the Greek meaning "to change shape," and that's exactly what metabolism is about, not only the transformation of raw fuel into usable forms of energy, but also the expulsion of waste products created by the burning of fuel. When we eat, our bodies take the basic elements of food (the macronutrients of protein, carbohydrate, fat, and alcohol), and through the digestion process transform them into forms of fuel our bodies can use. That fuel is transformed into energy by the cells. Metabolism consists on one level of the processing of raw energy (eating, digestion, combustion, and exhaust) and on another level, of cellular housekeeping. And it requires more than just calories to keep these interlocking and intertwined systems working—otherwise we could just eat candy bars all day.

But that's merely the physical aspect of it. There are countless psychological elements at work when we eat, many of which have little if anything to do with actual fueling or hunger, but most of which are equally as important to us as people. If we were machines, we could leave it at that.

For most of us, however, food is and should be a considerable pleasure. Meals are a time for enjoyment and for sharing that enjoyment (would romance even be possible without meals?). Many of us treasure our family dinners as a time to discuss the day's activities, refresh family bonds, and relax together in a pleasing environment. Certainly this can be seen as a replenishing of energy, but it is also a replenishing of the spirit, which is equally important.

Our pleasure in food has both good and bad aspects. One of the unique and wonderful things about being human that we can take from and give great pleasure and comfort with food. But if food becomes the only or central place we find comfort and pleasure, we run the very real (and all too common) risk of getting out of energy balance.

In addition to the minimum amount of calories we need to maintain BMR, each of us needs an additional but variable amount of energy to accomplish all of our daily physical tasks. A roofer, lugging heavy shingles up ladders and working in the hot sun all day long, has considerably different energy needs than someone sitting at a computer terminal.

Here's a pretty simple formula for energy balance: Average number of calories consumed minus average number of calories burned equals your energy balance.

We should exist in energy equilibrium, burning, on average the same amount that we consume. An increasing number of us, however, exist in what is known as a positive energy balance, which is to say that we consume more than we burn—and this is one of those cases where a positive is really negative. What happens to the excess? It becomes stored energy, and the form in which our bodies store most energy is fat.

Some people exist in a negative energy balance—but negative is only occasionally positive: if you're trying to lose weight or if it's a temporary state (energy restriction, as we shall discuss below, has some positive effects on cancer and other disease). If negative energy balance is prolonged, it becomes starvation.

In an ideal world, all of us after we reach full growth (around eighteen for women, around twenty-four for men), would maintain energy equilibrium. This doesn't mean we'd eat and burn the same number of calories every day. It means that over a given period of time, the calories we consume would roughly equal the calories we burn.

Using the tests and tables provided in the preceding chapters should give you a pretty good idea of whether over years or decades you've maintained energy equilibrium. How much did you weigh when you reached full growth? What do you weigh now? Unless you're a pregnant or lactating woman, someone who's been bodybuilding, stopped smoking, or were significantly over- or underweight at your age of full growth, are you about the same weight? Or have the pounds crept up on you? For example, over the last seven months you may have burned roughly the same number of calories you consumed. But if you gained twenty pounds between the time you reached your full growth and seven months ago, you may be at a higher risk for cancer (unless that twenty pounds is muscle). If this is so, then like a number of Americans, you may want to consider restricting your energy and spending some time on the negative side of the energy balance equation. This does not, however, necessarily mean you need to starve yourself or diet in the conventional sense.

Energy excess has been linked to cancers across the board. In several comprehensive studies, women who had the lowest risk for cancer had body weights ranging from 20 percent *below* average to 10 percent above. Obese women (defined as more than 40 percent overweight) were found to have a whopping 55 percent increased likelihood of *dying* from cancer over women of average weight. Obese men were found to have a 33 percent greater likelihood of dying from cancer than those of average weight. Lowest incidence among men was also found in body weights 20 percent *below* average to 10 percent above.

You can eat your way to better health *and* get into energy equilibrium by eating the same volume of food. What you change is the *quality* of the foods you eat by eating fewer and smaller portions of energy-dense foods and stoking up on nutrient-dense foods (which, by comparison, tend to have a much lower energy profile). We will discuss this concept in chapter 7, and we'll discuss energy foods and nutrient foods[15] in separate chapters in Part III.

energy restriction

The evidence indicates that if a body's energy supply is in equilibrium, if the body has a healthy ratio of fat to lean body mass (the body is fit and in the range mentioned above), and if the body's cells have adequate nutritional assistance to keep their natural, built-in defenses in top working

---

[15] The distinction made here between energy supply and nutritional supply is in some respects artificial: Energy is *part* of nutrition. But the distinction is important because most of our diets are energy rich and nutrient poor. Those foods that have a relatively low energy profile but a high nutrient profile (green leafy vegetables, for example) are those that are most important to have lots of in our diets to maintain top cancer health. In Part III we have therefore made the distinction between energy foods and nutrient foods, recognizing that neither is exclusive of the other.

order, then the energy we consume will be used by the body's normal tissues and processes. Cancer will, more often than not, stop before it starts. A key part of this equation is physical activity, which is the only reliable way to maintain that healthy ratio of fat to lean body mass.

In energy equilibrium, mutant cells that slip past the body's guard won't have as much energy available to develop. Energy equilibrium, then, is one of the most important aspects of stopping cancer before it starts. But animal studies (and some human research) have also indicated that *restricting* energy can seriously retard or halt cancer cell proliferation. Energy restriction also has positive effects on other disease as well.

Exactly why energy restriction—or feeding a body only approximately enough energy to maintain BMR, or basal metabolic rate—has such an effect on cancer is not precisely understood. Neither is it known precisely why energy *excess* has such a negative impact on cancer prevention. But the leading theories as to why both occur are tightly intertwined.

It is possible that energy intake controls cell growth. Metabolism is, from one aspect, the turnover of cells. The availability of excess energy may increase cell replication and thus cancer risk (the more times cells replicate, the more opportunities there are for cell replication to go awry). It is also possible that obesity makes for higher levels of chemical carcinogens stored in body fat. Excess energy may also lead to breast cancer by changing the turnover of hormones, some of which, after menopause, occurs only in the adipose or fat tissue.

There are other reasons why physical inactivity and obesity may increase the likelihood of cancer. Although it has not yet been conclusively proven, energy imbalance that leads to obesity may result in what you might call metabolic discombobulation, or a condition known to researchers by the mysterious-sounding label of "Syndrome X." The result may prove to be a physiological environment in which growth-promoting hormones are out of balance and growth is promoted generally and for tumor cells specifically.

So if all of this can occur with energy surplus, it doesn't take a great leap of logic to figure out that restricting energy might have opposite effects. But the unanswered question is why. There are several theories.

Our bodies have several growth hormones. One of them is insulin, which you may associate with diabetes. Insulin isn't just something that diabetics have to inject, it is one of the most important metabolic hormones: it builds tissue, but it's also an energy regulator. One of the tissues it builds is adipose tissue—fat. This is a good thing because without that capability we'd have no stored energy but the protein in our muscles and organs. But like so many good things, it's also potentially dangerous. All animal bodies need stored energy. We're not like lamps—you can't take a human away from its energy source and then plug it back in and expect it to work.

So insulin and its fat-building properties are necessary to survival—which is why Type I diabetics, most of whom no longer produce any insulin, will rapidly die without injections. But too much insulin can result in serious problems. One of them, apparently, is our old enemy cancer.

Insulin is made in the pancreas and stored there, then released when we eat. It maintains blood sugar at desirable levels by a variety of means. Some it delivers to the cells to be burned for energy; some it converts to a starchy substance that's stored in the liver, muscles, and other tissues for release when blood sugar drops; and the rest it converts to fat and deposits in the adipose tissues. But it also interacts with other growth hormones.

As noted in the previous chapter, a lean body is much more finely tuned, much more efficient—test an athlete and her serum (blood) insulin level will be quite modest. She doesn't need a great deal of insulin because she's quite sensitive to it. She's in energy balance and her systems are working the way they were designed to work. Test an obese, sedentary couch potato, and her serum insulin level will be comparatively quite high. She's out of energy balance and her hormonal systems are out of balance as well.

Again, the mechanism for why a slim body is so much more efficient than an obese one isn't precisely understood, but all over the body there are countless receptors for all sorts of chemicals, from neural receptors to hormonal receptors. When we overload our bodies, which many of us do on a regular basis, sensitive receptors get progressively desensitized or do what's known as down-regulate. This is precisely why a drug addict constantly needs to use more of the drug to get the same effect—because he's overloaded his receptors and they've down-regulated. The wonderful thing about the human body is that it's quite resilient and almost constantly capable of being resensitized, although permanent damage can be done.

One of the central theories about why energy restriction is good for us but bad for tumors concerns insulin. When you have lots of energy stored away in the form of body fat, there's plenty of energy for a tumor to grow on, and plenty of room for the body to store chemical carcinogens. But that's not all of it. When you have high levels of growth-stimulating hormones floating around in your system, they're going to do what they are supposed to do: stimulate growth.

Energy restriction appears to force the body to burn fat stores and process out those chemical carcinogens. Getting rid of the fat also resensitizes the insulin receptors (or up-regulates them). This allows for much lower levels of serum insulin and helps get the other growth-promoting hormones back into balance. If you feed a human or research animal higher levels of nutrient-rich but energy-poor foods, you also introduce all kinds of fiber into the gut, some of which assist in biotransformation in remarkable ways, carting off unwanted hormones and thereby preventing their return into the system but also carting off a variety of toxins.

As an example of how body fat affects growth hormones other than insulin, consider estrogen. Estrogen levels, you may know, are related to osteoporosis, the potentially crippling, progressive loss of bone density that can happen to women after menopause (and also, to a much lesser degree, to men, particularly after surgery for prostate cancer). Hormone replacement therapy, which seeks to restore the estrogen a woman's body no longer produces after menopause, is an effective means of preventing this loss of bone density. But it is also thought to be related to a somewhat higher risk of breast cancer. Interestingly, heavy women have a lower incidence of osteoporosis but a higher incidence of breast cancer. The reason would appear to be the interrelationship between fat and tissue-building hormones. As noted above, the conversion of some hormones into estrogen after menopause takes place only in fat tissue. Women who gain weight later in life, particularly after menopause, also have a greater risk of breast cancer. The reason is the same. Girls who have a high-energy diet as youngsters tend to reach menarche earlier than other girls; they also have a higher risk of breast cancer. Girls whose energy is restricted as youngsters (who are highly athletic, who eat a nutrient-dense diet, and burn the energy they consume) reach menarche later and have a much lower incidence of breast cancer.

Much research needs to be done yet on energy restriction and its mechanisms; clearly energy is necessary for life, but too much energy can be deadly.

the take-home message on cancer and energy

There is no evidence that there is any food that must be completely ruled out of your diet, unless you want to rule it out, have an existing medical condition, or use a particular medication that makes it necessary to avoid certain foods. Energy balance can be achieved best not by narrowing your diet but by exactly the opposite (this doesn't mean that you should therefore try every dessert on the menu). You should get as many different foods into your diet as possible, while also making certain you eat lots of cancer-fighting nutrient foods. After reading chapter 9, you may never look at your diet the same way. A narrow diet leads to chronic dietary patterns, and the research has shown that it is chronic dietary patterns, chronic energy surplus (night after night of empty-calorie desserts; months or years on end of little or no vegetables and fruits; lots of salted foods; nightly meals of fatty meats) that will increase your risk, not momentary indulgences.

Optimum health in terms of cancer prevention occurs for men and women who range from between 20 percent below ideal body weight to 10 percent above. Those who maintain fitness and this kind of body mass exist in energy equilibrium, or a neutral energy balance, and will have the lowest incidence and mortality of cancer.

If you're overweight or obese, the best way you can work towards this state is to center your meals and snacks on vegetables and fruits, reduce your portions of energy foods, and eliminate the chronic consumption of highly processed foods and meats.[16] Increasing your physical activity level as you do this is vital.

---

[16] As you will note in chapter 8, "meat" as the term is used here indicates *only* the commercially farmed red meats, beef, lamb, and pork, and does not include poultry, game meats, or fish.

part III

the best nutrition for cancer prevention

7

choosing to eat healthy

how to eat?

Intelligently.

But what does it mean to eat intelligently? Actually it's not dull or even especially brain-intensive, requiring a nutrition guide cracked open on the table next to your plate. That's homework—and if you find that pleasurable, then fine. But intelligent eating of an entirely different order is what culinary experts and gastronomes throughout the ages have recommended. Not eating to stuff yourself, nor merely to fuel yourself, nor to satisfy gluttony (although there are times when, as a special treat, you might want to go to that all-you-can-eat seafood buffet).

Intelligent eating nourishes body and soul, renews you with the breaking of bread. Intelligent eating is sharing with family and friends that same nourishment of body and soul, appreciating and understanding the most subtle and delicate delights food has to offer allowing contrasts in textures and flavors to overwhelm your senses. Intelligent eating is understanding your own pleasures and pursuing them, finding new and adventurous avenues for their appreciation and fulfillment.

Intelligent eating always includes at its root sensible nutrition, and makes sensible nutrition the basis for discovering ways to make food better—more interesting, lively, satisfying.

Intelligent eating is knowing what you're eating, and, in terms of your own biology, why you're eating it. Which is not to say that intelligent eating means discarding your comfort foods. It does mean, however, examining them: why are they comforting? How can you (if you want or need to) make them tastier, more nutritious and even more satisfying?

In the end, intelligent eating is about *quality,* about coming as close as possible to making each meal, each snack, a culinary masterpiece.

But, you respond, you're not a chef, not a nutritionist, not a culinary expert or gastronome! Nonsense. In a sense, we are all chefs, nutritionists, and culinary experts. Who is more expert on what you like than you? On what your family likes?

What may be a masterpiece for your husband's intimate fiftieth birthday dinner isn't necessarily a masterpiece for your daughter's soccer team's tournament victory lunch. Yet both can be healthful. Both can be delicious. Both can be pleasing to the senses. Both can be masterpieces, after their own fashion.

The best news you will find in this chapter—aside from the specific cancer-prevention guidelines at the end—is that you can pretty much include any of the many different possible foodstuffs in your and your family's diet (including the occasional "sinful" dessert), as long as you don't overdo the empty calories. The key word here is *occasional.*

More good news is that the things that are good for you really are *good* for you, and the things that are bad for you (unless it happens to be spoiled or bacteria-laden food) aren't all that bad for you, provided you stay in balance. What is "bad" for one person may be nutritionally appropriate for another—lots of protein may be just the thing for a growing teenager or a highly athletic adult, while completely inappropriate for an overweight, sedentary, middle-aged person.

Remember, eating for cancer protection or prevention is a balance, and how far you want to take nutrition to the lowest end of the risk spectrum is up to you. If you want never to eat sweets again in your life, that's a decision you can make, and you, your teeth, your waistline, and your health may be better off for it. But remember also that cancer risk is based on chronic dietary patterns, so if all other things are in balance, a holiday weekend of over indulgence in fat- and sugar-laden desserts is not likely to give you cancer or any other health problem. Do it every weekend and the story most likely will be different.

The body is highly resilient and can recover from an astonishing level of abuse (stopping smoking, for example, reduces your risk of heart disease almost immediately). But isn't it better not to abuse your body in the first place? Of course. The better your healthstyle in the first place, the better able to resist cancer and other chronic illness you're going to be.

paying attention to the nutrition of our ancestors

Our bodies evolved their built-in defenses because our ancestors were the survivors. Those who didn't have them would have died long before they could reproduce.

But our bodies did not evolve in a vacuum. The same is also true of plants. Indeed, long before we or our primate ancestors roamed the earth, the earth was covered in plants. Without plants, which themselves have covered the lower part of the earth's atmosphere with vital oxygen, we could not exist. No matter whether we eat animal or plant foods, all of what we eat derives its energy from plants and their interaction with the sun. Whether it's eating fish that eat bugs that eat plants, or consuming animals that eat plants—all of our food sources derive originally from plant forms. Photosynthesis is the process by which plants transform solar energy into energy that's useful to them. One of the by-products of photosynthesis is oxygen.

All plant and animal life are dependent upon oxygen: plants exhale it and animals inhale it. We utilize the oxygen that the plants produce in order to turn the energy sources we ingest (protein, carbohydrate, fat, and alcohol) into energy that's useful to us. We can't burn that energy without oxygen. But in burning oxygen, as noted previously, we create reactive waste, which, if not properly packed up and carted off with the help of antioxidants, can itself cause genetic damage. Prolonged exposure to sunlight, as most people know, can cause damage as well. It creates the same kind of reactive compounds. We can, of course, get out of sun and wear sunblock but plants are utterly dependent upon the sun, so it is not surprising that those plants that survived to reproduce were those that could protect themselves from the nourishing yet potentially harmful rays of the sun.

Those of our prehistoric ancestors who survived to reproduce developed, through coevolution with plants, ways of protecting their own bodies with the chemicals in the plants. So in a very real sense our bodies have particular metabolic expectations of our diet. This includes not only vitamins and minerals, which are vital, but other, less well known micronutrients. These micronutrients are known as phytochemicals, literally, "plant chemicals." If we don't meet our bodies' needs for these chemicals, which have only recently begun to be catalogued and understood, then our defense mechanisms can't work at peak capacity. The parts of plants that are most densely packed with phytochemicals are those that are metabolically active—the leaves and ripening fruits. The seeds, which consist mainly of energy stores (usually in the form of fats) and dormant genetic material, are not so rich in these chemicals, although they often have, as whole entities (whole grains, for example, which are the seeds of grasses), other valuable nutrients.

The human race and its evolutionary predecessors have roamed the planet for millions of years. Agriculture as we know it has only been with us for about ten thousand years, a blink of an eye in evolutionary terms. And given that there are still a few hunter-gatherer societies on the planet, it's a safe bet that not all of our ancestors converted to an agricultural diet ten thousand years ago. Which is to say that our ancestors came up on a diet considerably different from the one most of us consume today.

Yet if our forebears had such a great diet and we have such a lousy one, why do people of today live so much longer, and why do athletes of today continue to break records and barriers with astonishing regularity? The answers aren't all that complicated. We have much more reliable food supplies than they did, a much better understanding of how the human body works, much better medicine (much lower child and maternal mortality thanks to good prenatal and neonatal care), protective immunizations and antibiotics, and so on. And because of this better understanding of how our bodies work, our contemporary athletes can train better, eat better, and more thoroughly explore their absolute limits.

But don't think for a minute that the top athletes in the world have the same sort of diet as your average person on the street, or the same level of physical activity. As discussed earlier, obesity in this country (and in much of the developed world) is on the rise, and shows no signs of slowing. The sedentary lifestyle is epidemic in the United States, with as much as 80 percent of the population getting essentially no regular exercise at all—not even twenty minutes a day of walking or its equivalent. Try breaking any barrier with that kind of training. And when you consider that few of us eat the recommended average of five servings of fruits and vegetables a day, it's actually quite remarkable that we *aren't* in the midst of a cancer epidemic. But then again, in ten or twenty years, we may be.

Although no one can really say what we were meant to eat, we can deduce what works best from how our bodies are constructed. If we were meant regularly to eat such highly concentrated energy sources as refined sugars, or half a pound of meat (with all its saturated fats) at every meal, we would not need such a large gastrointestinal tract. If we were not meant to process the various types of dietary fiber that are so vitally important to health, we would not need the space for all of this undigestible material—nor would we have coevolved with so many friendly bacteria to help utilize this material.

To make more clear the kind of diet our evolutionary forebears might have eaten, imagine that your family and perhaps a couple other families become marooned together on an island. It's not a desert, but it is remote, has four seasons, and while there's food, you have to find it—there are no drive-in windows, no domesticated animals, no processed grains (no donuts or bagels or delivered pizza). Neither is there any processed sugar—no candy, ice cream, cakes and pies. Instead of driving to work, sitting at your computer all day, then coming home in the evening and popping something in the microwave to eat it while you watch the evening's TV lineup, you'd probably be spending a lot of time fishing, hunting for edible leaves, fruits, berries, tubers, and so on. If you ate meat, it wouldn't come in a foam and cellophane package; you'd have to hunt it. You'd also probably spend much of your time doing a lot of physical labor to maintain a place to live and sanitary conditions. Just washing clothes would be strenuous physical labor, but that would be the least of it. Your body would be forced to work hard and do so almost constantly. All the while you were finding food for today, you'd also have to be thinking about what you were going to eat in the winter, because this is not a tropical island. There would be times you would go hungry. If you became ill, you would not be able to do much hunting or gathering.

Consider these points:

◆ Most of what you'd eat would be the fruits and leaves of plants, with some fish and perhaps the odd game animal.

◆ The fish and game you'd eat would be quite lean, because it, like you, would not be feeding at a trough and standing in a barn all day but hunting and gathering.

◆ Your physical activity would be pretty much constant, although it would not necessarily be the same kind of intense, temporary exertion you'd experience in an aerobics class, training for a marathon or lifting weights. It would just be constant.

◆ Obesity, if it was a problem before you arrived on the island, would not be a problem much longer. There might be strings of days when you had little or no food at all.

◆ When it got dark, you wouldn't do much but sit around a campfire or sleep. But you'd need your rest because when the sun came up it would be time to hunt for food and gather berries, and so on.

In a very general sense, these conditions are probably much like those under which our bodies evolved. Constant physical activity. Lean times. A diet very high in vegetables, fruits, tubers, seeds, and perhaps whole grains. Protein would have come from plants, fish and game, and other very low fat sources.

What does this have to do with cancer? Consider these points:

◆ The human body has been shown to be much more efficient when its energy consumption is restricted (this is true of animal bodies in general—see below). Our bodies can be quite stingy with energy because over the millennia they had to be. But an energy-restricted diet doesn't necessarily mean one that's deficient. It just means that instead of filling up on energy-dense foods, you'd fill up on food that's much higher in a diverse array of nutrients that aren't found in those concentrated energy sources. (In the past year, how many different kinds of vegetables and fruits have you eaten? Some researchers estimate that our forebears probably ate, in any given year, a hundred or more different kinds.)

◆ Although precise mechanisms for *why* the body is more efficient are not fully understood, it makes sense that a certain amount of hunger should hone the senses. Those of our ancestors, who awoke in the morning with an empty belly but who were not mentally alert, probably didn't survive to very old age. If you hadn't the stored energy or the proper balance of hormones to release energy when needed, you probably wouldn't be able to muster sufficient energy to meet your body's caloric needs.

how much to eat?

Exactly how much you eat and what you eat are things you're going to have to decide for yourself based on your lifestyle, energy balance, and tastes.

The recommendations in this chapter are based on our increasing knowledge of how diet can profoundly affect cancer risk. The weights and measures are based on an average energy requirement of two thousand calories a day.

In many respects, two thousand calories a day is an arbitrary number, based on an average person who may or may not actually exist. Although your energy needs may indeed normally be two thousand calories a day, they may easily be more or less, and they may differ at particular moments in your life. You may need more of particular nutrients in your diet if you're recovering from illness, less if you are out of energy balance. You may need more if you're building up on a strenuous exercise program, such as training for a marathon, or less if you're recuperating after running your marathon.

So the point of having a number like two thousand calories is not to have you get out your calculator and the food value books and count calories for everything you eat in a given day. The point is to focus your attention on where most of your calories come from and where most of your cancer-fighting nutritional bioactive compounds[17] come from, and how these balance in the overall equilibrium of energy in your healthstyle. Are the elements of your diet proportionate to your needs and to one another?

making food whole again

Back in the 1960s, on those old futuristic sci-fi TV shows that now run endlessly on cable, a little door whooshed open and out came a little plate with

---

[17] Bioactive compounds, as noted earlier, are a broad category of nutrients that are biologically active. Some bioactive compounds, such as vitamins and minerals, are commonly understood. Others, such as phytochemicals, are not so commonly understood nor so readily categorized.

three or four different colored tablets, each perhaps representing a different food group, and that was a meal. The plate that held them was the anachronism, and the tablets themselves were perhaps the logical endpoint of the scientific research that went into NASA's freeze-dried space food packets. We had a lot of faith back in those days in the ability of science to distill things down to their essence, to take all of the important nutrients in foods and do exactly what science had done with pharmaceuticals. Certainly for many of us with our crammed days and hectic schedules, it might be convenient now and again to be able to down a few brightly colored tablets, consider it a meal, and keep on going.

We were right to have faith in science, but probably wrong to think that good science was necessarily the distilling of everything down to its essence. Food and nourishment, we have come to understand, are filled with far more important aspects of life and living than definable or extractable essences. Food means survival for the spirit as well as the body. Look at all the religious rites that center around food and drink. Jews give up food for Yom Kippur; Moslems give up food and drink from dawn till dusk during the holy month of Ramadan; for Christians, the bread Christ broke and wine he shared have become important sacraments among His adherents worldwide.

Food and the rituals of eating are integral to the spirit of our humanness, and that humanness extends from the spiritual into the physical and back again.

Our gastrointestinal tract is a big, hollow tube that was meant to be filled. And what's more, it has been shown that our bodies have the clear biological expectation that it will be filled with certain things. As we have said before, we did not evolve in a vacuum but in a world full of foodstuffs, and our bodies have what appear to be in states of optimal health when we are full of the foods we evolved eating. Many mysteries still remain about what we eat and how it affects us that may never be resolved. (The American Gastroenterological Association admits, for example, that it still isn't quite sure why stomach acids can break down dietary proteins so readily but leave the lining of the stomach—protein—intact.)

Despite the mysteries that do remain, it is clear that a good, cancer-protective diet isn't just a matter of getting your RDAs. The term RDA—Recommended Dietary Allowance—is used throughout this book, but you should be aware that the meaning of the term is not necessarily what it has traditionally been. New recommendations, called Dietary Reference Intakes (DRIs), are being developed by the Food and Nutrition Board of the National Academy of Sciences. DRIs identify average requirements of a population, maximum safe amounts to avoid toxicity, and RDAs. But as new RDAs are set they will be based not only on preventing deficiency diseases as in past editions, but to name nutrient levels that will promote optimum health (ie. preventive health concerns) for almost everyone. DRIs will eventually be set not only for protein, vitamin and minerals traditionally included, but also dietary fiber and a variety of phytochemicals. We absolutely need the many phytochemicals and other bioactive compounds that are increasingly understood as crucial to good health and to cancer prevention.

Because food is food and not pills or capsules or extracted, isolated nutritional components, it is best to talk about foods as whole foods rather than as the various pieces that may be found in them. It's important to know that such compounds are in them, but you don't have to know all of that because researchers are isolating new compounds in them every day. And although some have been researched exhaustively, there are many more that have not. So just because you haven't heard of a particular compound doesn't mean it's not good for you.

But there is some difficulty in talking about foods in a whole sense because most of the research into foods and their effects on disease has generally centered on individual compounds, the components within foods. This makes sense—a particular compound shows promise in reducing or preventing mammary tumors (breast cancer) in mice, so researchers look into the chemical to find out if and how it works. Many of our current medications come from just this kind of research. And it makes sense from a practical standpoint: Looking at a single compound is relatively simple; combining it with one or two or a hundred others (as might be found in a carrot or sweet potato, both fine sources of beta-carotene) creates so many variables that it makes an experiment almost impossible to control. Yet at some point and in some way, all of the variables have to be brought together.

In the following pages, while we look at the categories of foods, or food groups, we will look at different foods that are good sources of various nutrients, including vitamins, minerals, phytochemicals, and other bioactive compounds. But the most important thing to keep in mind as we do so is that eating a broad and varied diet of whole foods, rich in nutrients, is the best way we can reduce cancer-risk and optimize overall health.

food, glorious food!

Although there can be no such thing as a cancer-proof diet, the research is clear that there are many dietary practices we can put into play that will reduce our risk of cancer, reduce other chronic illness, and improve overall health. There really are almost countless different kinds of foods we can eat—some of which are more healthy than others, but nearly all of which, at some level, can be worked into a sensible, cancer-preventive diet. No book of this scope could possibly list them all with the good or harm they each might do. That would take a massive database that would expand daily as we learn more and more, and would have little practical value in helping us make choices at mealtimes.

We can, however, show you which *types* of foods do which kinds of things, and how by emphasizing or de-emphasizing particular nutritional elements in your diet you can reduce your cancer risk. We can also—and shall, as we go along—show you new ways of looking at your customary foods to make them tastier and more protective against cancer.

The wonderful thing about food in the nineties and beyond is that there are about as many possibilities as you can imagine. Food can be had year-round from the four corners of the globe—tomatoes from Holland, pineapples or crab meat from Indonesia, apples and kiwi from New Zealand, grapes from Chile, asparagus from Peru, berries from Guatemala, fish and even seaweed from Japan, and beef from Argentina, to name just a few.

A few years ago you could find one sort of banana in most groceries, the Cavendish banana. Today, you can often find plantains (bigger, firmer green bananas that are most often cooked), the small, oddly-named lady-finger bananas (which resemble the fingers of no lady we know), and even red bananas. (More on bananas later.) You can find plum, beefsteak, hydroponic, and even striped tomatoes, not to mention sun-dried. You can find a vast array of peppers, from sweet red and yellow to the hellishly hot scotch bonnet or habañero. You can find a dozen or more different kinds of rices, from basmati to wehani, some with the wonderfully nutty-tasting and nutritional germ and husk still attached.

Salad once meant iceberg lettuce (designated by some only an honorary vegetable for its relatively low nutritional profile) and maybe even Jell-O. But now you can find more different kinds of greens than you can count. And once you could get only white mushrooms, canned or fresh, or, if you were especially intrepid and didn't mind the possibility of poisoning, perhaps three or four more if you went hunting for them yourself. Now, in most groceries, you can get many different types, from the delicately fla-vored cremini and porcini to the silky-textured shitake to the big, meaty portobello.

There's also an enormous variety of potatoes—from pearly, white-fleshed baby red potatoes to the creamy, yellow-fleshed Yukon gold, to pur-ple and other multi-hued varieties. You can find even more exotic kinds of potatoes at farmers' markets or through specialty seed companies. And then there are daikon, jicama, tomatillos, quinoa, kasha, lemon grass, kiwi, starfruit, papaya, and all sorts of other "new" vegetables, fruits, and grains that have been popping up on grocer's shelves over the last several years. And don't forget all the wonderful herbs, packed fresh, that you only used to be able to get in little bottles as desiccated powders and leaves.

There are probably any number of reasons for the appearance of these new foods on grocery shelves over the last several years. Changes in immi-gration laws have changed the faces of immigrants, and many new Americans have brought their food preferences along with them—and some of these you will only find in small, ethnic groceries. Increasingly aware of the health benefits to be derived from fresh fruits and vegetables, consumers have demanded not only variety, but fresh, local produce when possible. And food producers have responded to the demand for what once were considered exotic foods by expanding their (and our) horizons.

Perhaps the biggest impact on the public hunger for exotic foods, how-ever, has been the proliferation of cooking shows on television. These have an effect a bit like that of sitting in a restaurant and watching someone else's meal go past and thinking, Hey, that looks *good.* The chefs travel all over the world, and even back in time, figuratively speaking, sampling recipes and wares of all sorts of different cultures, exposing their audiences to food and drink they never knew existed (or never dreamt they could make themselves).

Suddenly the old standard of hamburgers and french fries looks shabby and colorless, especially considering what we know about saturated fats and the potential for contamination. Couple that with a growing concern for the effects of cholesterol, charbroiling, and saturated fats, and you have the roots of a potential revolution in the way people in this country eat.

But let's not discount taste, either. Fruits and vegetables just plain taste good. The fresher they are, the tastier they are.

what you need to know

So with all of these choices, how do you know what to eat? We'll ask again: What do you *want* to eat?

We often talk about comfort foods, foods that comfort us because of our associations with them. Child psychologists say that one of the most stressful events in a child's life is facing unfamiliar food. Because children are bombarded with so many new sensory stimuli, kids want at least a few things to be familiar, and food is one of them. Being hungry and then being faced with something that looks weird or smells weird can really throw a child. Are adults that much different? In certain respects, probably not. But as we grow, we tend to tune out many of those stimuli that overwhelm kids, and our tastes expand and grow. Our to-die-for food at nineteen is probably not going to be our favorite food at thirty, and a favorite at thirty may not be at fifty. Most of us have learned through experience and experimentation that the new can also be the exciting and delicious, and by the time we're twenty-five, we may not even have tried what may become our favorite foods yet.

But we are creatures of habit, and there are many others of us who find the prospect of new foods discomforting and daunting—we go to a restaurant and order the most familiar-looking thing on the menu. This may also depend on mood as well. Some days you may feel like starting a four-alarm fire in your mouth with a bite of habañero salsa, while on others you may opt for the same comforting old pot roast. There's nothing wrong with either, but eating intelligently means trying to look at old foods in new ways.

One of the things we've tried to do in the recipe section at the end of this book is offer up new foods by taking many of the foods you are no doubt familiar with and looking at them in completely new ways. How do you make that boiled broccoli into the emerald treasure it can be? How about broccoli as a dip? Not as a part of a vegetable platter you dip into a bowl of fatty white goo, but the actual dip itself? Why not? See our Broccoli and Mustard Dip on page 229 for a completely new way of looking at this super vegetable. Or how about broccoli sprouts? Recent research at Johns Hopkins University indicates that broccoli sprouts have many times the suspected cancer-fighting chemicals of broccoli itself.

But how do we know what to eat for optimum cancer protection? What to make of all these foods, familiar and not? If there are so many it would take a never-ending database to update them all, how can we possibly know what's in all of them and what's not—and how good they are for us?

In one sense, we can't—not even the most up-to-date researcher could tell you every last bioactive compound[18] that occurs in, for example, a single carrot. But in another, more important sense, it's actually pretty easy to talk about this vast array of different foods in a way that's sensible, helpful, and informative. Eat all of them. Research shows that the more consistently varied your diet is, the healthier it is likely to be. Surprise yourself.

In practice, you don't *need* to set up your diet with one eye on the RDA chart and another on the food labels. You can eat intelligently and enjoyably without knowing every last bioactive compound and phytochemical[19] in your food. You don't absolutely *need* to know, for example, the nutritional breakdown of an orange—that it contains vitamin C, carotenes, and other valuable antioxidants, but no vitamin B_{12}—although knowing won't hurt you.

What is probably more important for each of us to know rather than the breakdowns of individual foods are the basic categories of foods—the food groups. If the term makes you think you're in for the same old thing, worry not. We've taken a considerably different angle on food groups than the one you'll find in the Food Guide Pyramid. Although the general idea is similar—encouraging you *not* to eat a monotonous and potentially deficient diet—our breakdown of the categories will prove much more informative about why we eat the kinds of foods we eat, and how improving our intake of certain kinds will also improve our health. Our approach shows you how to make choices within the various categories and subcategories—knowledge that can help improve your health.

So what do you need to know?

---

[18] A bioactive compound is one that can be digested or otherwise utilized by the body (certain kinds of fiber are undigestible, but still bioactive). Many of the bioactive compounds we derive from food can be quite healthful, while others can be poisonous or carcinogenic.

[19] From the Greek, meaning literally "plant chemical." See "Phytochemicals and Bioactive Compounds," in chapter 9.

the essentials of your diet

You need to know where your energy and your nutrients come from, and what the *quality* of your energy supply is. Are your calories loaded with nutrition or are they empty?

You also need to know that whatever makes up your diet, there are certain essential[20] dietary components you must have:

- adequate essential amino acids (amino acids are the building blocks of protein)
- adequate essential fatty acids (fatty acids are the body's negotiable currency of lipid, or fat, and used for a variety of purposes, including the construction of cells)
- essential vitamins and minerals
- enough calories to provide fuel for all your activities and body processes

It helps, also, if you know where to get them—which we will explain. While you must have these things to survive, surviving by itself isn't living well.

There are other dietary elements that may be essential to your health that are not yet entirely understood. In a sense, the evidence is increasingly clear that there are many nutrients that we need for good health for which the recomended amounts—at least as far as conventional RDAs are concerned—simply don't exist. These include such things as antioxidants—crucial for cancer protection but not yet well-enough understood for there to be a scientific consensus on how much we might need, and exactly what kind.

There are also elements of our diet from which we do not get energy or even nutrients in the conventional sense, yet these dietary essentials work in our bodies in other ways to help keep us in balance and cancer healthy. This "nonnutrient nutrient" subcategory includes the various kinds of fiber.

The research is clear that beyond the accepted RDAs there are many other things we not only need but our bodies expect—and statistically speaking, many of us are simply not providing our bodies with them. It may be that in the future we will have RDAs for compounds that only cutting edge researchers have heard of today.

---

[20] An essential nutrient is one that cannot be synthesized by the body and so must be consumed in the diet.

taking another look at the food guide pyramid

The government's *Dietary Guidelines for Americans*—which is available for free to anyone who wants it, and which includes the Food Guide Pyramid—is an extremely good, basic source of information about diet and nutrition. The dietary guidelines are designed to help answer the question: What should Americans eat to stay healthy? It provides advice about food choices that promote health and prevent disease in healthy Americans aged two years and over.

Yet despite the ubiquitousness of the Food Guide Pyramid—on cereal boxes, bread wrappers, in school lunch rooms—many people aren't clear on how to translate it into real food choices.

Some of it may have to do with the idea that you can—and should—break down foods into servings, sort of like breaking down paper money into coins that can then be exchanged, ten of these for five of those. If this is the only way you have of measuring such things, then it's probably better than nothing. But it also leaves a good deal to be desired, because, for example, trying to turn a piece of lasagna into its respective servings of the

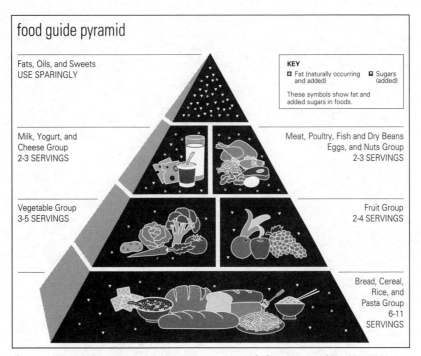

Source: The U.S. Department of Agriculture and the U.S. Department of Health and Human Services.

grain, milk, meat, and vegetable groups, then do the exchanges, and come up with a sensible notion of how many servings you've just had and from which group is more than a little daunting. Even on a simpler level, one slice of bread is not the same as another. Take a look for a moment at the government's graphic, "What Counts as a Serving?" A slice of bread counts as one serving from the grain products group. That's fine as far as it goes, but a thick slice of very dense seven-grain bread may weigh four or five times what an ordinary piece of white or wheat bread does—all of which takes you into unknown territory. Have you had one or two servings? Or three?

Now take a look at the fine print at the bottom of the servings table. Some foods are "crossover" foods and can be counted as servings in more than one group. But a crossover food can't be counted in one group if you're counting it in another. (Dried beans, by the way, have a considerably

what counts as a serving?*

GRAIN PRODUCTS GROUP (BREAD, CEREAL, RICE AND PASTA)
- 1 slice of bread
- 1 ounce of ready-to-eat cereal
- ½ cup of cooked cereal, rice, or pasta

VEGETABLE GROUP
- 1 cup of raw leafy vegetables
- ½ cup of other vegetables—cooked or chopped raw
- ¾ cup of vegetable juice

FRUIT GROUP
- 1 medium apple, banana, or orange
- ½ cup of chopped, cooked or canned fruit
- ¾ cup of fruit juice

MILK GROUP (MILK, YOGURT, AND CHEESE)
- 1 cup of milk or yogurt
- 1½ ounces of natural cheese
- 2 ounces of processed cheese

MEAT AND BEANS GROUP (MEAT, POULTRY, FISH, DRY BEANS, EGGS, AND NUTS)
- 2–3 ounces of cooked lean meat, poultry, or fish
- ½ cup of cooked dry beans, 1 egg, two tablespoons of peanut butter, and ⅓ cup of nuts each count as 1 ounce of meat.

*Some foods fit into more than one category. Dry beans, peas, and lentils can be counted as servings in either the meat and beans group or vegetable group. These "crossover" foods can be counted as servings from either one or the other group, but not both. Serving sizes indicated here are those used in the Food Guide Pyramid and based on both suggested and usually consumed portions necessary to achieve adequate nutrient intake. They differ from serving sizes on the Nutrition Facts label, which reflects portions usually consumed.

different nutritional profile than fresh, canned, or frozen vegetables, and do not cross over in our recommendations.)

All of this, while it may at heart be sensible nutritional advice, leads to a lot of unnecessary confusion and calculation.

Currently, for many of us, a serving of meat might be a quarter to half a pound, while a cup of raw leafy vegetables (one serving) may be all the green vegetables we're likely to eat this week—despite the fact that the leafy green vegetables may be the healthiest food we'll eat all week long.

And while the central goal of the Food Guide Pyramid is to promote a healthful, balanced diet that includes all the essential nutrients to prevent disease and deficiency, as well as an appropriate level of energy, judging by statistics it does not seem to have its desired effect. America grows increasingly obese. Children are more and more sedentary, obese, and hypertensive. A recent survey reported that only 1 percent of children two to nineteen met all the government's recommendations for a healthy diet. Chances are pretty good that these eating patterns reflect those of their parents. The children surveyed may actually be more honest in reporting their dietary intake than their parents, the parents being wise to what they are expected to say (or what they wish were true) rather than admitting the reality.

Whatever the worthy foundations of our food pyramid, there is no reason why you have to be part of the statistics—that three-quarters of our population that don't even come close to eating adequate amounts of vegetables and fruits.

the food categories

For our purposes in this book, there are two main categories, energy foods and nutrient foods, and each includes a spectrum of foods. The energy foods include a higher ratio of the macroconstituents of our diet (those things you can see) to micronutrients (those things you'd need a microscope to see), while nutrient foods contain a higher ratio of micronutrients. Neither category, of course, is mutually exclusive. Energy foods contain nutrients and nutrient foods contain energy. But we go to each category for its strength. Meat,[21] for example, an energy food for its protein and fat content (both are nutrients), is also a good source of iron, selenium, and zinc, but we eat meat mainly for its protein.

Although our categorization of foods is quite similar in many respects to that of the Food Guide Pyramid (and our basic advice of eating a primarily plant-based diet is very much the same), it's really more like a food family tree than a pyramid. Our interest is in informing you of what you can eat (and avoid eating) to minimize your cancer risk and improve your overall health.

The point of grouping foods at the top as either energy or nutrient is primarily to help illustrate the differences in the ways that energy can and should be balanced. While you certainly need both energy and nutrient foods in your diets, if at meals and snacks, you're eating primarily energy foods, you might be eating foods that will increase your cancer risk while ruling out foods that could decrease your cancer risk. You may also, in this way, be maintaining a positive energy balance, thereby increasing your risk. Potato and corn chips, pretzels, and candy are all nearly pure energy with a very low ratio, by weight, of nutrients, fiber, and so forth. If you're eating these snack foods at every snack and not burning the calories, then this is going to throw you towards the unhealthy side of the spectrum. Conversely, fruits and vegetables such as carrots, broccoli, celery, and apples will have a much higher ratio of fiber and nutrients to energy, and if you eat these regularly as snacks, they will push you toward the more protective end of the spectrum. And they will just as readily fill you up.

So by categorizing foods in this way, we can show you quite simply how you can substitute similar quantities of nutrient foods for energy foods and improve your energy balance while simultaneously improving your health.

Our food groupings will give you more thorough information on what the kinds of foods we eat do for us—the difference between empty calories and those that are loaded with nutrients, for example—as well as how ratios of these foods can easily and tastily be arranged and adjusted to fit into your healthstyle.

Overall, the best reason for categorizing foods this way is to explain and expand upon the recommendations that appear in chapter 11, giving specific dietary reasons for the recommendations, including many of the stud-

---

[21] *Meat* as the term is used here includes domesticated, farm-raised red meats: beef, pork, and lamb, and excludes game, fish, and poultry. Game will tend to have a much different fat profile from domesticated meat, although farm-raised game (such as venison), which is growing in popularity, should probably be considered as meat rather than game because it too will have a much higher level of saturated fat (which is why it may taste better than wild game to some people).

ies that have gone into the construction of the recommendations. Why, for example, is alcohol not recommended for *anyone?*

Certain of our groupings may surprise you. Even though we categorize fruits as nutrient foods, we do not include bananas, perhaps the world's most popular fruit, as a fruit even though bananas (and other plantains) are, botanically speaking, fruits. Their energy and nutrient profile makes them fit much better with the energy foods of roots and tubers, and in many parts of the world, they are eaten as starchy staples rather than fruit.

Each of the following sections is broken down along the spectrum of these food groups, describing pluses and minuses, and exploring how each may affect cancer risk.

This is all pretty simple information, easily put into practice, with lots of suggestions on how you can make your eating more intelligent, more pleasurable, and more healthy—all without trying to figure crossovers or exchanges. While we want you to think about what you eat, we don't see any point in forcing you to make such calculations.

8

energy foods

The word *energy* derives from the Greek for "active," and so energy foods are the foods that provide us with fuel—zip, bang, power. Energy foods are those that will give us most of our calories. Let's now talk a bit more specifically about energy and calories and the kinds of foods that provide us with our daily energy supply, and about the different qualities of energy.

It's worth mentioning that heat itself is not energy but the evidence of it, just as expensive clothing or jewelry is not wealth, only evidence of it. Energy, or the potential for work, is actually sort of complicated (it is a law of physics that energy can neither be created nor destroyed, only transformed). For our purposes, think of it this way: When you go about work, whether it's exercise or just maintaining your basic metabolic rate, you heat up (or stay warm). The heat you experience is the evidence of calories being burned, the evidence of energy use or transformation. Where the human body is concerned, there is one other notable evidence of energy use, and that's the transformation of potential energy into its storage form: fat. You eat, and it's either burned, or you get fat. Pretty simple.

the energy foods, by category

The nutrients which categorize energy foods are:

- **fat** (the most energy dense at about 9 calories per gram or 252 calories per ounce)
- **alcohol** (more energy-dense than carbohydrate or protein at 7 calories per gram or 196 calories per ounce. Alcohol should not be a significant source of energy for most people.)
- **carbohydrate** (4 calories per gram or 112 calories per ounce); and
- **protein** (roughly equivalent energy density to carbohydrate, at 4 calories per gram or 112 calories per ounce, but considerably different in its metabolic activity and function)

calories

If you're a food label reader and have ever wondered where the number of calories for a particular food—a candy bar, a fish stick, a frozen dinner, or even a bottle of soda—comes from, it's calculated by a process known as calorimetry, which is a fancy way of saying, calorie measuring.

As you know, a calorie is a measure of heat, and so the process of finding out how much heat a particular food can produce—and therefore how many calories it contains—is simple: you burn it. Everything your body burns can also be burned by fire, and that's exactly how calorimetry works.

If you've ever burned a steak or a roast or had a pie drip in the oven, you know that some things can burn hotter (and with a lot more smoke) than others. Others hardly burn at all. Your oven may still be giving off whiffs of that tuna casserole that overcooked back in 1973.

Calorimetry is, of course, a much more controlled process than a dripping pan in the oven, but it's easy to see that all of the energy foods can, at least when compared to nutrient foods, produce a *lot* of heat. If you happened to drop a few leaves of spinach in the oven, you might not even notice when they went up in smoke—unless they were attached to a quiche.

Indeed, most of the things we burn as fuel for our bodies can also be burned as fuel for heating, lighting, and other purposes. Fat and alcohol, with their high energy density, are the best sources—oil in lamps, and so on. However unappetizing it may seem to us, people in many developing countries use animal dung as heating and even cooking fuel. There are locales in this country where grain is more plentiful than timber and you can have your wood-burning stove outfitted to burn corn. The heat produced is substantial.

But just because a food contains calories doesn't necessarily mean your body will utilize them. And not all calories are utilized at the same rate or in the same way. The more basic the form—fat, sugar, simple, processed starches—the more readily the potential of the calories to be converted to energy, burned, or stored away as fat. (Consider, for example, that whale oil burns much more efficiently in an oil lamp than the actual whale.) The more complex a food is, the less easily the energy it contains is transformed. This is good, in a sense, because energy must be used simply to access the energy.

This is knowledge you can use to your benefit not only when trying to maintain energy balance or drop a few extra pounds, but also just in general when trying to improve your health and reduce cancer risk. As we will discuss in the ensuing sections, it may be true, as Gertrude Stein said, that a rose is a rose is a rose, but overall, it is not the case that a calorie is a calorie is a calorie.

the qualities of energy foods

To give you a broad idea of how different one calorie can be from another, consider that you could run a calorimetry study on a pine two-by-four, the kind of lumber you might find in the frame of your house. You'd find a lot of calories—a lot of potential energy. But the key word here is potential. If you ground that two-by-four down into sawdust and could somehow manage to choke it down, what would happen? You'd have a bellyful of sawdust and your body would unlock next-to-none of its energy potential.

Why?

Each of the energy foods is made up of particular kinds of building blocks—proteins of amino acids, fats of fatty acids, and carbohydrates of saccharides. The bioavailability of the energy locked in the food is dependent upon the body's supply of enzymes with which to unlock these building blocks and convert them into bioavailable compounds. Think of it as a little like currency exchange—British pounds are not legal tender in the United States, as is the dollar. If you take them to a currency exchange and convert them into dollars, you can spend them anywhere.

And so despite the number of calories resident in a two-by-four, they wouldn't become energy because the human body simply hasn't got the enzymes to turn those calories into energy. (Curiously, even termites haven't the enzymes to break down cellulose—they're dependent upon their own gut flora to break wood down into bioavailable energy.)

Although you'll probably want to leave two-by-fours out of your diet, knowing that a thousand calories from a donut are not the nutritional equivalent of a thousand calories from quinoa tabouleh, can minimize your cancer risk and help you eat smarter. The point here is that calories come in many different kinds of packages, and in at least one sense, the packaging of the energy is as important as the energy itself. Unlike commercially pre-pared foods where packaging is just trash, with whole foods, their endoge-nous packaging is often the most nutritionally rich part of the food. In a general sense, the more of that natural packaging (the germ and bran of grains, the skins of vegetables and fruits) we eat, the better.

utilization of energy foods

So how do we know which foods our bodies utilize more readily than others?

While burning foods can give a pretty accurate measure of how many calories they contain, measuring how many of those calories are actually absorbed by the human body is another thing entirely (and not something you're likely to see on food labels). First, absorption of calories will likely vary from body to body—if you're accustomed to eating certain foods, you may have a more ready supply of particular enzymes to break down those foods. This is another example of the up-regulation and down-regulation we discussed earlier. Eskimos, who traditionally get less than about 10 percent of their diet from carbohydrate (from berries in summer), have such down-regulated supplies of enzymes for breaking down carbohydrate that when they're exposed to starchy or sugary foods, they can experience extreme stomach upset, including diarrhea. The popular saying "use it or lose it" has a fair amount of validity when we're talking about various bodily functions, although it should be noted that the body is remarkably resilient, which is why it is possible for a thirty-five-year-old sedentary housewife to turn herself into a heavy duty triathlete in a few years' time—and for the Eskimos to learn how to digest carbohydrate.

So if food's calorie content is relatively easy to measure—you just burn it—how do you figure out how the body utilizes it?

That's pretty straightforward too, if a little more involved.

To simplify somewhat, the researcher would feed a particular food with a known value of calories to a research volunteer (more likely several volunteers, and probably several times, in order to establish averages). The intrepid researcher would then collect the volunteer's waste products and run a calorimetry study upon them. By subtracting the remaining caloric content of the waste product (what's left over after the body has extracted what it wants or needs—e.g., urine and fecal matter) from the original caloric potential of the food, the researcher would then have a pretty exact idea of how many calories the intrepid volunteer had absorbed from that food.

If you're wondering, *What on earth are they doing with those research dollars?,* this kind of study is extremely useful in finding out not only how resistant to digestion certain foods are, but how compounds in the same foods are almost completely digestible and others almost completely undigestible. White rice, for example, is a low waste food—it's almost completely digested. So if you're burning a lot of calories—out in the fields or down in the mines working all day—white rice is a great food. If you're essentially sedentary, the energy conversion of any excess calories is not going to be into work, but into body fat. This doesn't mean that white rice is bad for you, it's only an example of how 90 to 100 percent of the measurable calories of one food might go straight into the energy supply while only 40 to 50 percent of another food might.

There are other values to this kind of research as well. Analysis of the contents of the waste products, not just for remaining calories but also for leftover vitamins and minerals, hormones, and residues from the kinds of flora that grow in the gut, as well as the balance of all of these things, tells us a lot about cancer risk. Certain kinds of dietary fiber, for example, will absorb metals, while others will sop up (or bind) bile acids, fats, as well as excess hormones. Knowing in general that fibers do these jobs is important to knowing how to eat the right kinds of things to reduce cancer risk.

Knowing that particular packages of energy provide not only energy, but many other nutritional, metabolic, and health benefits, while other packages of energy don't, can enable you to take the foods you like and engineer your own cancer-healthy diet.

Reading the basic information (which is very basic) on food labels is a good start to finding deciding are healthy foods, and which are foods you might want to leave alone.

carbohydrate

Carbohydrates can take on a pretty astonishing variety along the spectrum from simple to complex. From table sugar to your favorite bread, from the veggies in your salad to the flowers that decorate your table to the very table itself (if it's made of wood), carbohydrates are everywhere.

Since carbohydrates—in the form of starchy staple foods such as cereals (grains), tubers (potatoes, yams, etc.), and plantains (plantains, bananas, etc.)—should, according to our guidelines, make up about 45 to 60 percent of your energy supply, it makes sense to talk about carbohydrate first. And since cereals (grains) will make up the largest portion of that, it makes sense to talk about them first.

Cereals are the processed seeds of cultivated grasses, from those you're highly familiar with such as wheat, barley, oats, and corn, to others with which you may not be so familiar (and may not even be able to find in your supermarket), such as teff, millet, sorghum, quinoa (pronounced KEEN-wah), kasha, and bulgar. The ways cereals can be and are eaten are almost infinitely variable: You'll find cereals in everything from your fried chicken to your candy bar.

So while you may not think of pasta or pastries or corn chips or tabouleh as cereal, that's exactly what they are. And all of them are processed or refined to some degree, even if that processing only means removing the wheat from the chaff. Cereals are remarkably versatile, and in terms of health, that's as much a mark in their favor as a mark against them.

do carbohydrate energy foods increase cancer risk?

Studies throughout the world suggest that diets high in sugars may contribute to an increased risk of cancer of the colon and rectum. There is some evidence that pancreatic cancer risk may also increase, but evidence is really too sparse to judge.

On the other hand, diets high in (dietary) fiber are associated with a decreased risk. The evidence here is stronger, ranging from the pretty-close-to-conclusive (high levels of dietary fiber are shown again and again to reduce the risk of cancers of the colon and recturm although no one can say without a doubt, "eat fiber and you won't get cancer") to the possible (even though the evidence is inconclusive) regarding a possible protection by fiber against breast and pancreatic cancers.

Diets high in fiber have been thought since the 1960s to be protective against colorectal cancer. In its 1982 report, the National Academy of Sciences noted that some individual studies had found links between starch-rich foods and an increased risk of cancers of the esophagus and stomach, and between sugar and an increased risk of cancers of the pancreas and breast. While interesting, the NAS's judgment at that time was that the information was too meager to allow for any firm conclusions. That same report noted links between fiber intake and a decreased risk of colorectal cancer, but found this information to be inconclusive as well. The dietary guidelines issued as part of the report did, however, emphasize the value of whole-grain cereals.

The 1988 U.S. Surgeon General's report on nutrition and health examined a mass of evidence published in the 1980s that suggested that fiber-rich foods protected against colon cancer. Although the evidence was inconclusive, the Surgeon General recommended increased consumption of whole grain foods and cereal products. A 1989 report of the NAS, noted human and animal studies suggested a relationship between sugar and breast cancer and recommended consumption of more complex carbohydrates, breads, and cereals, and limiting sugar consumption. These recommendations were based more on other diseases (such as cardiovascular disease) than cancer.

In 1990, the World Health Organization recommended that 50 to 70 percent of total energy in diets should come from complex carbohydrates, noting that such diets "seem to favor a lower incidence of a variety of cancers," and also recommended that consumption of dietary fiber be between sixteen and twenty-four grams per day.

Like everything else when we talk about dietary macronutrients and cancer, carbohydrate exists along a spectrum. No single type of carbohydrate is likely to *cause* cancer, but certain types consumed in large quantities over a long period of time to the exclusion of others are likely to increase the likelihood of many cancers. Most expert reports distinguish between starches and dietary fiber on the one hand, and refined sugars on the other—so-called complex and simple carbohydrates. When the AICR/WCRF expert panel reviewed the one hundred such reports published between 1961 and 1991 (which were mostly concerned with diet and cardiovascular disease or diet and chronic disease generally in the developed world), they found that sixty-two recommended more starch or complex carbohydrates, with none disagreeing; sixty-one recommended more fiber; and seventy-four recommended less refined sugar, with none disagreeing.

the take-home message on carbohydrate and cancer risk

In order to lower cancer risk, limit refined sugar and starch, while eating more whole grain foods and more vegetables and fruit.

simple and complex carbohydrate

You may have heard distinctions made between simple and complex carbohydrate, but if you're like most people, you may not be entirely sure what the difference is.

In certain respects, dividing up carbohydrate this way is helpful, because it allows us to pick and choose between what might be called fast-acting and slower-acting carbohydrate energy foods. But in other respects, the common distinction between simple and complex carbohydrate is really a false—or perhaps incomplete—distinction.

Carbohydrates are *polymers*, or complex compounds formed from other molecules. In the case of carbohydrate, those other molecules are saccharides, or sugars, which are themselves made up of carbon, hydrogen, and oxygen—a formula that sounds a bit like rocket fuel—bonded together in different combinations.

Like other polymers, these sugar/starch molecules consist of chains, some with branches, some without; the number of molecules and the shapes in which they are chained determine the kind of sugar or starch they are, as well as the kinds of enzymes necessary to break them down.

Dietary carbohydrate comes in four main types (whether from cereals, roots and tubers, plantains, or from nutrient foods):

- mono- and disaccharides, or simple sugars
- polysaccharides, or starches[22]
- oligosaccharides,[23] or starches that are mostly undigestible
- and nonstarch polysaccharides (NSP), usually thought of as fiber or bulk

The simplest, shortest chain carbohydrates generally taste the sweetest. These are the mono- and disaccharides, or single or double sugars. Glucose, or the kind of saccharide the body uses as blood sugar (and one of its primary currencies of potential energy), is a monosaccharide, as is fructose, or fruit sugar. Table sugar, on the other hand, is sucrose, a disaccharide, and is made up of a glucose molecule bonded to a fructose molecule.

There are many other disaccharides, but most of them have one thing in common with monosaccharides and many polysaccharides: The calories in them are almost instantly available to your body as energy. That is, they will give up glucose or energy when exposed to your body's enzymes. This giving up of glucose molecules begins almost immediately upon putting food in your mouth (saliva itself being full of enzymes) and continues through the stomach and into the small intestine, where most of the extraction of energy and nutrients takes place.

The more complex a carbohydrate is, the more reluctantly it gives up glucose and the harder it makes the body work to break down the saccharide chains. If the starch and sugars in a particular food are enclosed in the cellular structures of the whole grain, or are bonded to longer chain carbohydrates, the calories in them are turned into burnable fuel more slowly. Carbohydrate foods that break down more slowly will tend to stay in your

---

[22] Polysaccharides are often referred to as complex carbohydrates, but many of them are as fast-acting in terms of energy as simple sugars.

[23] *Oligo-* is a prefix that means "few," and the way it's used in describing carbohydrate means that the oligosaccharides are made up of only a few (three to ten) saccharides, but are irregularly shaped and "give up" few of their mono- and disaccharides in digestion. Although they are not thought of as fiber, they are also undigestible for the most part, and it is from these undigested oligosaccharides that gut flora really go to town and create gas. Not surprisingly, they are plentiful in legumes, but even more plentiful—and gassy—in other foods, most notably, raw apples, bananas, raisins, cooked cabbage, and onions. Despite the occasional embarrassment of gas (which can be controlled with a preparation such as Beano), they are good for you and quite desirable in a cancer protective diet.

stomach longer, leaving you feeling fuller. But—conversely—as they reach the bowel, they tend to move along more rapidly. Many of the calories you consume may not actually be turned into energy, but into other valuable cancer-fighting bioactive compounds as your food passes into the large intestine from the small.

Think of it a little like firewood: Big fat logs burn slowly, releasing heat over a longer period of time; split them into kindling and they'll burn hot and fast—you will get a hotter fire quicker, but the fire will also go out faster. Best is a mixture—a little kindling to get the fire going, then some larger logs to keep the fire burning and providing heat. Processing and refining in a sense is the dietary equivalent of splitting cereals down into kindling—but you need the big logs, as it were, to keep you going.

While we eat energy foods for energy, those which tend to those give up energy over a longer period of time are generally likely to be of a better *quality* of energy, as well as better for your health. There are several reasons for this. Foremost, if food stays in your stomach longer, the less likely you are to experience hunger pains and eat more, whether you need it or not. This is what's known as your sense of satiety.

A word on satiety, or the feeling of being not hungry after eating. An example of satiety, a kind of satisfaction, would be when you sit back and say, "My, that was delicious," but not, "I'm stuffed." Different kinds of foods will give you different sensations of satiety. You could eat, for example, three hundred calories from fat or three hundred from complex carbohydrate. The complex carbohydrate will probably give you more of a feeling of satiety than the fat for the simple reason that it is less dense and more filling. Satiety also has to do with occasion. If you're just a little hungry at your desk during the long hours between lunch and dinner and want a snack, eating an apple will probably give you a sense of satiety. If you've been out running eight or ten miles, it may take more—a bowl of oven-baked onion soup, a plate of salmon cakes, and a slice of sweet potato pie—for you to achieve a sense of satiety. The thing to keep in mind with satiety is that it's a *feeling*, and may not have anything to do with your dietary or energy needs.

While satiety is important, the largest part of the nutrient value of carbohydrate foods tends to reside in the cellular structures that make up the bran and germ of the grain. And it's not just vitamins and minerals, which tend to be concentrated in those structures, but the fibers themselves that are crucial to reducing cancer risk and enhancing the cancer-protective quotient of your diet.

Learning how to adjust the kinds of carbohydrate you eat to get more complex carbohydrate and less refined carbohydrate isn't difficult, doesn't take willpower, and isn't like eating sawdust.

It's really not complicated. The point here is knowing that reading the Nutrition Facts labels on the products you purchase can provide you with good information on the different qualities of carbohydrates in the foods you buy—but it helps to know what you're looking for. Generally, the more processed or refined a food is, the fewer kinds of carbohydrate and fiber tend to be present in it. In the most highly refined foods, such as cakes and white breads, cookies and most packaged breakfast cereals, there may be little but sugar and simple starches.

So, while we want to get a substantial portion of our dietary energy from carbohydrate, we also want to make certain that it's the right kind.

processing, or how to know good carbohydrate from "bad"

It's important to take a moment to talk about refining or processing, because it's processing that most often is going to make the most difference between the quality of energy to be had in cereals. Most cereals are about 70 percent starch by weight; the other 30 percent is where most of the micronutrients and fiber resides. In refining—and all cereals will be processed or refined to some degree—it's that 30 percent that gets removed. Even boiled rice is often milled to remove the bran and husk— and yet it's in the husk and bran that most of the nutrient value of cereals reside (to name just a few: iron, manganese, niacin, pantothenic acid, phosphorus, potassium, riboflavin, and thiamin). You needn't worry about remembering all of those various bioactive chemicals—just remember that empty calories means foods from which all or most of these good things have been removed.

Think back to that pine two-by-four we talked about earlier—eat the same weight of white rice and almost every bit of the calories in it will become available to your system. This is because you have the enzymes to break it down. Fine milling of starch products (as in making flour) disrupts the plant cell walls, and starch is often gelatinized[24] during food processing, so that it becomes similar in its metabolic effects to sugar, which is to say that it's more readily turned into energy.

---

[24] If you've ever used flour or cornstarch to thicken a sauce, you've seen gelatinization at work: The

Is this a bad thing? Again, the idea of good and bad isn't particularly useful. The more processing done outside of the body—either by the manufacturer or by you yourself in the kitchen, the more easily the starch is converted into energy in the body, whether you happen to need it or not.

Most of us in our culture, with our relatively low level of physical activity and often sedentary jobs, don't need lots of energy fast. We do, of course, need energy. But for most of us, it's much better for energy balance and health if the calories are absorbed slowly—or, in some cases, not at all, but passed on through the stomach and small intestine to the large intestine.

So when you're eating cereals, try to eat mostly grains that are as minimally processed as possible. For sandwiches, go for whole grain breads. For breakfast cereals, go for oatmeal, barley, or kasha, or go for meusli, which tends to be sweetened with fruit such as dates and raisins, rather than granola, which tends to have a lot of added simple sugar. Or make your own meusli from the grains you like. For side dishes, try bulgur or kasha or brown rice (or even wehani rice, which is delicious and still has the nutty bran attached). If you're making your own breads, instead of using all white flour, substitute some oat flour (a great source of soluble fibers), whole wheat flour (a great source of bran's insoluble fiber), and so on. The same thing goes for pie crusts and crumbles.

But if you're going to make a birthday cake, don't try to make it whole wheat—unless that's what you happen to like. And go ahead and have that donut after church. The idea is to make sure that the largest part of the cereals you eat on a weekly or monthly basis is going to be loaded with cancer-fighting goodies rather than empty calories.

To get an idea of how processed or refined a cereal product is, you can read the Nutrition Facts labels on the products you purchase and compare the amount of total carbohydrate listed to the total dietary fiber amount. The higher the ratio of dietary fiber to total carbohydrate, the higher quality nutrition you're going to get with your carbohydrate energy food.

How does this work? Try this experiment:

To demonstrate the way different kinds of carbohydrate actually work on the body, you can use yourself as the intrepid lab rat.

Try this for breakfast or for a snack, or whenever it's convenient. What

---

heating of the starch bursts whatever cell structure remains, releasing the starch and forming a gel. This released starch is much easier for the gut to absorb as pure energy. If you ate cornstarch straight out of the box (not that you'd want to), it will be—because of this gelatinizing process—digested quite differently.

you're going to do is eat two of the same type of food, one highly refined, the other minimally refined, on two separate occasions. Then decide which one gives you more of a sense of satiety and sticks with you longer.

First, choose your weapon: if you're a breakfast cereal lover, go for breakfast cereal. If you're a cracker-lover, go for crackers. For simplicity's sake, we'll use crackers as our example.

Go to the grocery and find two kinds of crackers. So the experiment is entirely about carbohydrate, make sure they're both fat-free. Find one type that's as highly refined as you can and another that's as minimally refined. How will you know? Take a look at the ingredients and the Nutrition Facts label.

Buy both types of crackers.

As far as our experiment goes, don't pay too much attention to the list-ed serving size. Your own serving will be of your own devising. You should use the serving information to figure out how many calories your own serv-ing will have.

For the experiment's sake, let's say you choose two hundred calories (what matters is consistency, not size), or whatever you feel would leave you with a feeling of satiety after your snack. If it takes you four or eight servings of the minimally refined cracker to get to the same number of calo-ries for a single serving of the highly processed cracker, fine.

You'll conduct this experiment over two days. Decide when you're going to have your experimental snack, and have it at the same time both days. If you have cracker #1 at 10:00 AM on the first day, then have cracker #2 at 10:00 AM on the second day. If your snack is mid-morning, try to have the same breakfast both days so that you will be equally hungry both days.

On an empty stomach, eat your crackers. Don't spread anything on them—that will ruin your results. If you need something to wash them down with, and you might, drink water. It doesn't matter exactly how much water you drink.

Note the time, then eat your crackers. Your snack should give you a sense of satiety—you should feel satisfied by the food you've eaten and not hungry. You don't have to be stuffed. Now go on about your routine. When you begin feeling hungry again, note the time and see how long it took—one hour, two hours, whatever.

Repeat the same procedure the next day with cracker #2.

The first thing you're probably going to notice is that the volume of higher fiber/minimally processed cracker #2 seems significantly greater—it may not be all that much heavier, but it will likely be bulkier—than cracker #1. To achieve your sense of satiety, you may find yourself not even eating the whole serving. You may also note that the minimally processed cracker doesn't taste as sweet, and you also may note that even if it's not salty, you're going to want more water. There is also the possibility that the duration of your snack—how long it takes you to eat these crackers—will be longer, but maybe not.

Again, note when you started eating. (If you're not accustomed to eating fiber, your body's enzymes may be down-regulated and you might, if you're eating a large amount, feel a little bloated.) When you start to feel hungry again, note the time.

Your results: Without your even doing the experiment, we can tell you what the results will be: Your sense of satiety will last a lot longer with cracker #2, your minimally processed cracker, than with the highly processed one. Why?

fiber: it's not just bulk anymore

From the discussion above, you know that it is from the mono-, di-, and polysaccharides that we get most of our energy from carbohydrate. These are chains that the body can break down readily and turn right into energy. So if the others are undigestible, why do we want them in our diet? If they're not supplying us with nutrition, what's the point?

While dietary fiber was once thought of as merely fiber or bulk, and pretty much beneficial in the diet because it absorbed water and helped keep things moving (an important function, associated with any number of beneficial effects, not the least of which is preventing constipation and the various sorts of damage it can cause to the bowel. But thanks to the groundbreaking epidemiological studies by D. P. Burkitt in Africa and around the world in the 1960s and '70s, as well as the work of many others in the field, it is clear that we can no longer look at fiber as a single, exchangeable entity. Fiber plays numerous roles, many of which directly impact our risk for cancer. As long as we're getting adequate energy in our diet, the greater variety of undigestible fiber we can get, the better it is for lowering our cancer risk.

So if fiber isn't just fiber, what is it and why is it good?

here is some news we bet you didn't know

Since the gut flora[25] have so many different and important and healthy functions in the body, they can be viewed as a sort of collective vital body
organ, with a flexibility and potential for metabolic transformation compa-
rable with, if not greater than, that of the liver. Imagine not having a liver.
And yet most of us consume so little fiber (nutrition authorities maintain
that only about a fourth of Americans get adequate dietary fiber) that we
are depriving ourselves of a vital bodily organ.

At least one researcher has said that a Nutrition Facts label that reads:
"Dietary fiber, 5 g" is about as useful as one that might say, "Vitamins, 5 g."
In other words, dietary fiber is so crucial to protection against cancer that
there are likely to be RDAs or DRIs of the particular kinds of dietary fiber
one day. At the moment, however, the research on fiber is relatively new,
and very difficult to distill into neat equations, but certain facts are clear.
Researchers have yet to sort out all of the intricacies of the effects of each
kind of fiber and each kind of gut flora—this difficulty partly being due to
the vast number of different kinds of bacteria that coevolved with us and
coexist in our large intestine, and the vast differences (because of dietary
differences) between the levels of these bacteria in different people.
However, just because things haven't been completely sorted out yet
doesn't mean that there is not already sufficient evidence to link cancer
rates to consumption of these different kinds of dietary fibers.

So what does fiber do?

Some pretty astonishing things, really. For example, in one study of
genetically similar mice, half were given an antibiotic that would annihilate
all the flora (bacteria) in their guts, rendering them germ-free. The control
group was not given the antibiotic. All of the mice were fed a compound
extracted from ferns that was a known carcinogen. What was also known
about this carcinogen was that gut flora that fed on a particular kind of fiber

---

[25] Gut flora are the wide variety of bacteria we have co-evolved with over the millennia that live
mainly in the large intestine and that work synergistically with our bodies in many different
ways. (One of the reasons antibiotics can cause diarrhea is because they kill off these beneficial
flora.) A few of the better known gut flora are those found in active yogurt cultures, such as l. aci-
dophilus— which is one of the reasons it's a good idea to eat yogurt if you get diarrhea. But there
are nearly countless others. A diet rich in vegetables and their constituent fibers promotes
healthy gut flora.

in the mice could detoxify the carcinogen. Those that were germ-free after the antibiotics developed cancer; those whose gut flora were left untouched did not.

This is pretty clear evidence that proper gut flora can neutralize certain carcinogens. And while that was a lab experiment and the variables were thoroughly controlled, there are studies on humans that show corollary results.

A study of American women vegetarians compared the levels of estrogens in their stool to that of a similar group of women who ate the common western industrialized diet—low in fiber, high in protein, fat, and refined sugars. The vegetarians eliminated as much as three times more estrogen than their nonvegetarian counterparts, and their blood levels of the hormone averaged about a third less. You should probably be able to guess from our discussions already why is this a good thing. But here's at least a part of the explanation:

Estrogen is the female hormone, but it is also an anabolic steroid, or a hormone that builds tissue (the anabolic steroids that bodybuilders use are often souped-up synthetic versions of male hormones, which build muscle mass rather than breast or ovarian or endometrial tissue). A healthy, premenopausal female body needs a certain level of estrogens, and all other things being equal it produces what it needs and eliminates what it doesn't want. Particular kinds of dietary fiber apparently evolved over the millennia as the body's exit ramp for excess hormones.

If the fiber isn't there to absorb the hormones (which happens in the large intestine), then the hormones hang around until they are reabsorbed and recirculated through the body. Excess estrogen can then cause unwanted tissue growth that could include cancer growth in the ovaries, breasts, and other female tissues. Excess estrogen is also a problem in men (because even though it is the female hormone, it is present in men, but in much lesser concentrations), and has been implicated in prostate cancer. It could be possible that it also plays a role in increased levels of breast cancer in men.

In addition to helping the body rid itself of unwanted hormones, fibers help the body eliminate excesses of bile acids (linked to cancers), cholesterol, alcohols, metals, and vitamins. And, as shown in the experiment with mice, it aids in the detoxification of potentially carcinogenic compounds. In some cases, fiber actually creates nutrients we need.

Vitamin B$_{12}$ is an example. Gut flora feeding on and fermenting or otherwise transforming particular kinds of fiber produces most of the B$_{12}$ we need.

You may be able to take supplements of vitamins and get all the B$_{12}$ you need, but by eating a diet that's fiber-poor, as most of us do, it's a bit like putting your metabolic trash collectors on permanent vacation. The waste just hangs around and your body becomes a toxic dump. So, clearly, getting sufficient dietary fiber can help us increase our protection against cancer as well as improve overall health.

soluble and insoluble fiber

Although our largest quotient of dietary fiber is made up of non-starch polysaccharides (NSP), there are, as you have no doubt guessed several different kinds of fiber. NSP is insoluble fiber.

If you took a big glass of water and dropped in a spoonful of each of the different kinds of dietary fiber and stirred them up, the insoluble fiber would sink to the bottom, while the soluble fiber would turn to something about the consistency of jelly. Insoluble fiber will absorb water—and whatever happens to be dissolved in the water—but it will still be visible in your glass of water. (Wheat bran is an example.) Pectin, the stuff that makes jelly gel, is one of the soluble fibers. (*Fiber?* you say. *But it's smooth.* Yes, fiber.) Perhaps you remember those containers of mucilage kids used to use in school for gluing together their art work—they have that rubber tip with the slit in the end and you press it down on the paper and squeeze out the mucilage. That, too, is a soluble, dietary fiber. Dietary fiber also contains lignin. When you eat a pear or lima beans, you experience lignin, which is what gives those foods their slightly grainy texture. Lignins are the only type of dietary fiber that isn't carbohydrate. They're also polymers, but they're made up of alcohols instead of sugars. They come from the woody parts of plants (that two-by-four would be loaded with lignins) and legumes, and are desirable in the diet because, among other things, they have antioxidant properties and can bind in the colon with bile acids and metals, preventing their reabsorption.

Each type of fiber is important, and each plays a different role in cancer health. What is clearest from epidemiological studies is that Americans as a group do not get enough of either.

so where do you get it?

FIBER	GRAIN	FRUITS	VEGETABLES	EFFECTS
Cellulose	Bran whole wheat whole rye	Apples, pears	Beans, peas, cruciferous vegetables, roots and tubers, fresh tomatoes	Insoluble; absorbs water; aids bowel motility; binds minerals
Non-carbohydrate fiber: lignin	Whole wheat, whole rye	Strawberries, pears, peaches, plums	Mature vegetables, legumes, woody portions of plants	Insoluble; has antioxidant properties; binds bile acids and minerals
Hemicellulose	Bran, cereals, whole grains	Apples	Beets, artichokes, corn, potatoes, legumes	Largely insoluble, some soluble; holds water; adds bulk to stool and aids motility; binds bile
pectins,		Apples, bananas, citrus fruits, berries, especially strawberries	Green beans, carrots	Soluble; binds cholesterol and bile
gums	Oatmeal, guar		Legumes	Soluble; binds cholesterol and bile; slows stomach emptying; fertile material for colonic flora
mucilages	Thickeners in prepared food products			Soluble; slows gastric emptying; fertile material for colonic flora; binds bile
algal substances	Thickeners in prepared food products	Algae, seaweed	Gums used in processed foods (carrageen)	Soluble; slows gastric emptying; fermentable; binds bile

the other starchy staples

We've spoken mostly about cereals up until now because they make up the largest portion of our carbohydrate energy foods. But there is considerable energy to be had from other kinds of carbohydrate energy foods: roots and tubers (potatoes, sweet potatoes) and plantains, such as bananas.

What's true of cereals is also mostly true of these other types of carbohydrate energy foods: the less processed, the better. The skins and the parts of the food close to the skin tend to contain the highest levels of dietary fiber and nutrients (but we don't recommend eating banana skins).

Cooking tends to release simple starches, and added fats often accompany cooking. French fries, potato chips, and fried plantains are cooked in oil or tallow; baked potatoes and sweet potatoes (at least in this country) tend to have fats such as butter, margarine, cheese, and sour cream added to them at the table or on the stove; sweet potatoes often have added butter, margarine, or sugars. See the recipe section for suggestions on how to cook with reduced levels of added fats and sugars.

As a group, roots and tubers tend to be good sources of NSP, carotenoids, vitamin C, potassium, other vitamins and minerals, and bioactive compounds.

so what is a serving, anyway?

You had to ask. From any sensible aspect, the notion of a serving can be complicated.

The recommendations for caloric consumption in this book are based on averages—as noted before, the mythical average American needs about 2000 calories a day to maintain energy balance.

If you're to get half to two-thirds of your average daily calories from whole grains and other starchy staple foods, that means you'll want to eat somewhere between 1,000 to 1,350 calories per day from those foods. Since carbohydrate offers about 112 calories per ounce, that means you'll eat about 12 to 16 ounces of carbohydrate energy food on average per day. This is an average, so it does not mean you must have exactly that number each day, only that, say, over a two-week period, you get about 28,000 calories from all of the foods and drinks you consume.

But these are just numbers, not whole foods, so the question remains, what's a serving?

In one sense, the idea of a serving is just this side of meaningless. An artfully rendered serving of *haricots vert* at the most *très chic nouvelle cuisine* restaurant is likely to be considerably different from a serving of green beans at the corner diner. There is no agreed-upon standard rating for serving or portion that everyone seems willing to accept. Rarely does any food come in a serving, as defined by the Food Guide Pyramid, or by food labels on most prepared products. How many servings are in a 20-ounce bottle of soda? One, but that's likely not what the label will say. In a nearly-half-gallon Big Gulp of soda? One.

If a package of sausage links contains eight links, why is three a serving?

What you want to know is *how much to eat,* and this is something you're going to have to decide for yourself, based on your body mass index, your energy balance, your physical activity levels, and your own good old common sense. We can talk numbers all day long, but if the numbers don't translate into real foods when you get into the kitchen, what good are they?

If 2,000 calories is your mark, then you have to figure out how to get your average 45 to 60 percent of starchy staples. If thinking in terms of standardized, defined serving sizes helps, then by all means divide up your foods into servings. If servings make no sense to you, then forget them.

A bowl of kasha or oatmeal or rolled barley—a serving—for breakfast might offer a quarter of that amount. If you add sugar or honey, that's instantly going to displace a larger quantity of higher quality energy. If you eat packaged breakfast cereals, you can use the food labels to help you figure out how much you're eating and how much fiber and highly processed carbohydrate you're getting.

Two slices of whole grain bread for lunch might make up another quarter. Forget the chips (which will add fat and lots of salt and not much in the way of food value). Add a banana, and you've probably got about three or four more ounces of carbohydrate energy food.

If for supper you have a serving (two or three tablespoonfuls) of Potato Gratin (see page 290), that could round out your allotment of starchy foods for the day. Again, if thinking of such things in servings is the easiest way for you to go, then go with it. If not, forget the idea of servings and just remember to eat plenty of plant-based foods, and then eat plenty more.

the take-home message on servings of carbohydrate energy foods

Many of us are creatures of habit and have a repertoire of foods that we cycle in and out of our weekly menus. Many of us eat exactly the same thing for breakfast or lunch, only getting variety at supper time. Instead, try to vary the food you eat throughout the day. If you're a breakfast cereal eater, try to eat a number of different kinds, and try to make certain that they're as minimally processed as possible—oatmeal on Monday, shredded wheat on Tuesday, and so on.

If you've been eating the same ham and Swiss cheese sandwich on white bread every day for the last seventeen years, introduce some variety, even if only in small steps. Try substituting a true whole grain bread (again, read labels) for the white, and use mustard instead of mayonnaise (there are lots of different kinds you can get). Pile your sandwich high with antioxidant-rich tomatoes, and leafy greens or some of the many different kinds of sprouts currently available. Or, for a complete change of pace, pack yourself a salad in one of those big plastic containers as part of your lunch. Use as many different kinds of greens as you can, add some sliced tomatoes, cucumbers, carrots or other veggies, and use a few dashes of flavored vinegar, low-fat bottled dressing, or just plain old lemon juice for a dressing.

For supper, try substituting bulgar or kasha for white rice or mashed potatoes. Have Quinoa Tabouleh (page 267) surrounded by lots of vegetables and a piece of broiled fish.

protein and fat

Protein energy foods are often linked to fat in the diet, and so it makes sense to talk about these two important sources of energy together.

Both protein and fat are essential nutrients—that is, each provides us with particular nutrients we cannot live without and which the body cannot manufacture from other sources. While a high-fat diet might eventually lead to cardiovascular disease or cancer, a no-fat diet would lead to deficiencies and kill you much quicker. The same is true of a no-protein diet. And fats and protein tend to work together in the body—cell walls, for example, are made from proteins and lipids. They work together with both positive and negative results for your health, depending on the quality of your energy intake and your energy balance.

But at the same time, they are considerably different in the way they provide us with energy, in the way they can be modulated in the diet, and in their quality and potential for cancer risk.

Since—after water—we are mostly made from proteins, let's talk about protein first, what it does and where it comes from, and how protein energy foods affect your health.

protein

In the same way that carbohydrate is not just carbohydrate but a host of different building blocks, so it is with protein. In this case, the building blocks are amino acids that our bodies break down and rebuild or synthesize as they need. Far from being "just protein," proteins are complex molecules that can be made up of as many as several thousand amino acids.

The framework of our bodies is made of stable fibrous, insoluble proteins. These include bone, cartilage, tendons, hair, and nerve fibers. Our muscles, organs, enzymes, peptide hormones, blood (hemoglobin and albumin), and milk (casein and whey proteins) are all made up of what are known as semisoluble, contractile proteins. But our bodies' utilization of proteins and their building blocks, amino acids, doesn't stop there. Individual amino acids also serve as precursors, or building blocks, for a range of crucial metabolic tools such as neurotransmitters, pigments, amines, nucleic acids, and various cellular metabolites.

Proteins are in constant flux in the body, usually as amino acids—always in use, breaking down in one place and rebuilding in another by means of hormones and other chemicals (also largely composed from amino acids, with a lot of help from lipids, or fats).

Our bodies are astonishingly resourceful when it comes to utilizing, manufacturing, and recycling proteins. Nearly all of the amino acids our bodies utilize are synthesized within the body from our various dietary proteins. There are, however, eight amino acids (nine in infants) our bodies cannot create from scratch. These are known as essential amino acids, and they are the collective reason any of us would die in short order on a protein-free diet. National agencies now stress that in most mixed, nutritional-ly-balanced diets (which, again, doesn't necessarily mean a low cancer-risk diet), most of us get sufficient essential amino acids regardless of whether they happen to come from plant or animal protein foods. Some dietary experts have in the past cautioned that vegetarians may not get sufficient dietary essential amino acids, but it is entirely possible to get all essential amino acids without ever eating meat.

The eight essential amino acids are: isoleucine, leucine, lysine, methio-nine, phenylalanine, threonine, tryptophan,[26] and valine. Histidine is the ninth, and some authorities maintain that all growing children should have it in their diet—but again, this shouldn't really be a problem for anyone eat-ing the types of foods common to the American diet.

If getting adequate essential amino acids isn't a problem, then our real concerns are first, how much of a part should protein in general play in your diet? and second, how will your protein intake affect your cancer health?

First, let's talk about protein and cancer risk.

does protein increase cancer risk?

The effects of dietary protein on cancer risk are so intimately entangled with the effects of other dietary macronutrients, particularly fat, that it's difficult to sort out exactly what—if any—effect dietary protein intake itself has on cancer risk.

First, there's the fat question—virtually all common dietary protein has some fat component. Some protein foods, as we shall see, have exponen-tially more calories from fat than from protein.

Second, there's the energy balance question, because the central char-acteristic of the typical Western diet is that it's high in protein, fats, sugars,

---

[26] You may recollect that the FDA banned the sale of l-tryptophan supplements several years ago after some consumers were poisoned by tainted supplements. The poisonings were not the result of the amino acid itself, but of poisons that were introduced into supplements at a single manufacturing plant. While there is some remote possibility of consuming potentially toxic lev-els of some amino acids when taking them in supplement form, that same possibility exists in taking dietary supplements of any bioactive compound—vitamins, amino acids, herbal prepara-tions, etc. Unless you have a condition or are on medication that inhibits your body's ability to process amino acids you should not, if you follow our dietary guidelines, need supplements, and you should run no danger of toxicity. See the recommendations on supplements at the end of the section.

salt, and simple starches, and rather weak in many of the cancer-healthy nutrient foods that will modulate cancer-risk downward.

But there's also the question of storage, preparation, and preservation of protein foods. Salting, smoking, added preservatives, and certain methods of cooking protein are all associated with a higher incidence of cancer. So, too, is spoilage.

Since protein rarely occurs in the diet alone (at some level, it is in nearly every ordinary food we can eat), in many respects it's possible only to make inferences and guesses about its effects on cancer risk. There is some inconclusive evidence that meat protein foods may increase cancer risk, and there is some slightly more conclusive evidence that protein foods from vegetable sources may decrease cancer risk. As with carbohydrate energy foods, protein foods exist along a spectrum. Also, as with carbohydrate, what affects the quality of protein foods and whether they might increase or decrease cancer risk probably isn't the raw protein itself but the nutritional components that accompany it.

Except in supplement form, the individual amino acids that are the building blocks of protein virtually never occur by themselves in foods, so it would be quite difficult to fashion sensible experiments that would tell researchers what, if any, particular amino acid might increase or decrease cancer risk. Still, it is possible to look at particular amino acids and know with reasonable accuracy what they do, and also to look at foods we know are high in, for example, lysine or tryptophan, and try to analyze their possible effects on health. But the many variables make concrete conclusions very difficult.

The National Academy of Sciences 1982 report, *Diet, Nutrition and Cancer,* reviewed evidence available at the time for cancers of the pancreas, colon and rectum, breast, endometrium, prostate and kidney, and concluded that although there was some evidence to suggest a role for protein as consumed in the United States in the genesis these cancers, it wasn't sufficient to draw any firm conclusions.

A 1989 NAS report concluded that evidence of a connection between protein intake and colon cancer was inconsistent (maybe it plays a role, maybe not). For breast cancer, that report found that dietary protein, especially animal protein, showed some correlation with increased risk, but case-control studies showed no *convincing* association. For other cancers, the information was limited—there is some evidence to suggest an influence of protein intake on pancreatic and prostate cancer, but the studies were few and there was little evidence for any other cancer sites. (It should be said that the protocols for scientific studies—or the mechanics and logistics of the manner in which they are conducted—can differ markedly from study to study, and in drawing conclusions from numbers of studies, the AICR panel, like any other group of scientists, had to look at these differences and try to balance them against one another—most often a difficult and complex task.)

As noted previously, all of our bodily tissues are made up of proteins, as is much of our bodily chemistry, and since cancerous growths are also bodily tissues that use bodily chemistry, they are also constructed from proteins. Yet just as, for example, eating protein doesn't automatically build muscle (you have to exercise to do that), neither is eating protein automatically going to build cancerous masses. We do know, however, than an overabundance of energy, regardless of its source, apparently feeds cancers. And it is the job of our genes, as the geneticists say, to code for a protein, or cause a protein to be made. Since, as previously discussed, cancer can be seen as a disease of energy and genetic material gone awry—the effects of protein on cancer and health cannot be ignored, no matter how difficult it may be to analyze its effects.

Some of the evidence considered by the AICR-WCRF Expert Panel in developing its report, and the recommendations upon which this book is based, included:

Lab animal experiments: In animal studies, low protein intake has been shown to inhibit cancers while high intake has been shown to promote cancer of various sites. (This may be as much a matter of energy restriction as of protein intake.) Most if not all animals used in a laboratory setting grow at considerably higher rates (and have considerably different metabolism and turnover of amino acids) than humans. Think of the old concept of dog years. At thirteen or fourteen, most dogs are quite old. A human of a similar age is still considered a child, and most often won't have finished growing by that point. Mice, rats, and other rodents have a far shorter life span, and since their genetic coding for protein use is so different, it's nearly impossible to apply such findings to humans in a *conclusive* way.

Preservation, preparation, and processing: Most meats have a high percentage of fat—often as high as 50 percent of their calories or more. Of this fat 50 to 90 percent can be saturated fat. While many of the processed meats you can find at your grocer—ham or roast beef, for example—may have much of the fat removed (some can be as much as 97 to 99 percent fat-free) others, such as bologna and hot dogs, can be loaded with fats. Despite their lowered fat profile, if you read the Nutrition Facts label, the salt content of packaged meats can be astronomical, which is a concern for cancer risk.

In addition, in order not to add fat in the kitchen (and improve flavor), many of us have taken to grilling meats. Indeed, grilling has become increasingly popular not just in the United States but all over the developed world for precisely these reasons. The problem with grilling, particularly over charcoal, is that many of the chemical by-products of grilling are known carcinogens or thought to be chemicals that can increase cancer risk. Evidence from various epidemiological studies shows a possible increase in the risk of stomach and colorectal cancer in diets high in meats cooked at very high temperatures—in other words, grilled.

While smoking was once necessary as a method of preservation (the smell of smoke scares off all kinds of microbes and bugs), these days we mostly smoke foods for flavor—smoked salmon virtually melts in your mouth, while a slow-smoked Texas brisket can, for some people, be almost a heavenly taste treat. In addition to flavoring meats, it can also add known and suspected carcinogens. Burned meat, in particular, should be avoided. Frequently, smoked fish, for example, is partly dried by adding salt before being smoked. This makes the naturally flaky flesh hold together better when it's subjected to the temperatures of smoking.

Does this mean you should completely avoid smoked, salty, or burned foods? If you want to stay at the very lowest end of the cancer risk spectrum—you could avoid these kinds of foods entirely. But cancer risk is based on *chronic* dietary patterns, not occasional indulgences. If you have smoked, salted salmon or burned brisket every day, it could increase your risk of stomach cancer. But if you have it as an occasional delicacy, it likely won't affect your long-term cancer risk.

Protein and other dietary macronutrients: As noted above, dietary protein (including that from vegetable sources) seldom arrives on its own, but is often accompanied by fats. As we in this country tend to get most of our dietary protein from animal sources, most of the associated fat is of the saturated variety, the kind most strongly associated with cancer and cardiovascular disease risk. The energy content of an egg, for example, is about 65 percent fat. Of that, 30 to 35 percent is saturated. We'll talk more about the difference between saturated, monounsaturated, polyunsaturated, and trans-fatty acids later in the fat section.

the take-home message on protein and cancer risk

While it cannot be said that protein causes cancer, there is evidence that diets high in animal protein do carry an increased risk of cancer. This probably has more to do with what accompanies the protein (fat) and what does not (diets high in animal proteins and fats also tend to be much lower in fruits and vegetables). There is also the issue of positive energy balance. Most of us get much more dietary protein than our bodies need, so our bodies have to do something with it. It can be converted into glucose by certain hormones, but if we take in more calories than we burn that blood sugar will end up stored as fat. If we can limit dietary protein to the necessary levels and increase the ratio of vegetable protein to animal protein we consume, the evidence shows that we will also decrease cancer risk and improve health. And if we can—at the same time—increase our intake of nutrient foods with their astonishing array of cancer-fighting phytochemicals and other bioactive compounds, and their lower energy profile, there is no question that we can move to the healthier side of the cancer-risk spectrum.

protein: how much you need, and where you can get it

For adults in the United States, the daily RDA for protein is 0.8 grams of protein for each kilogram of body weight. The recommended upper limit is about twice that level, or about 1.6 grams per kilogram of body weight (we'll show you below how to figure this out in pounds). This works out to about 10 to 20 percent of total calories coming from protein.

Current research shows that most Americans who follow the standard Western diet get considerably more protein than the recommended amount. This can present problems, especially when the source of that protein is foods from animal sources. While red meat, for example, is certainly a good source of protein, it also supplies saturated fat, and high intakes have been associated with an increased risk of high cholesterol, high blood pressure, and heart disease, as well as cancer. Just as important, as noted elsewhere in this book, the more of your daily calories that you get from sources such as meat, the fewer of your calories will be coming from high nutrient plant foods.

Although animal proteins are sometimes thought to be of higher quality than plant proteins, the reality is that all plant proteins are made up of the same combination of the same essential and non-essential amino acids. Not all plant proteins are equal, however; some plants have more of one essential amino acid and too little of another. That's why the best advice is to eat a variety of plant-based foods each day in order to get a mix of all the important amino acids.

But can plant foods supply sufficient protein in the diet? The answer is a definite yes. In fact, on a per calorie basis, most vegetables provide a higher percentage of protein than animal foods. The percentage of protein in plant-based foods such as legumes, broccoli, spinach, or mushrooms is about the same, or even a bit higher, than the percentage of protein in a broiled hamburger or a glass of low-fat milk. A plant-based diet that includes a variety of foods and meets your energy needs is also more than capable of providing sufficient amounts of protein for good health.

So how much protein is enough? The calculation, should you care to do it, is fairly simple. Just multiply your body weight by 0.36 and the answer is the recommended amount of protein that you should be eating each day for good health. Where did that 0.36 come from? Since a kilogram is about 2.2 pounds, 1 pound of body weight is approximately 45 percent of a kilogram. Thus the RDA of 0.8 grams of protein per kilogram of body weight becomes 0.36 grams of protein per pound of body weight when you multiply it by 45 percent.

Of course, the math isn't the important thing. Just multiply you weight by 0.36 and you'll have your recommended daily protein amount in grams. For a 125-pound woman, that would equal about 45 grams of protein. For a 180-pound man, the figure becomes about 65 grams of protein. If you are over- or underweight, just multiply your "healthy" weight by 0.36 (extra body fat does not raise protein needs).

If your likestyle includes a lot of physical activity, you may feel you need a level of protein somewhat on the higher side. But actually, while athletes building muscle through weight training may benefit from slightly more protein than the RDA, too much protein will lead to a positive energy balance, a higher intake of dietary fat, and a diminishing of other aspects of your diet. If you're filling up on steak or sausages or chicken, are you going to have room for broccoli, spinach, kale, and all those other super nutrient foods?

Rule of Thumb: four grams of protein per 11 pounds body weight.

some tables

The following tables are not designed so that you can paste them up on your refrigerator and refer to them religiously as though they were handed down from on high. They're here for illustrative purposes to compare different sources of protein and take some of the guesswork out of how you're eating, and help you eat more intelligently.

The government has recommended for years that we not consume any more than 30 percent of our energy from fats, but how many of us have any real idea of our true fat intake? Unless you're a nutritionist or a doctor, it's unnecessarily difficult to figure such things out precisely. And in truth, absolute precision here is not so important as being aware of what kinds of foods contain which kinds of nutrients, and how adjusting these can help you easily and painlessly adjust your intake to optimize your health and lower cancer risk.

These tables also offer a comparison between the protein and fat content of the protein energy foods so you can see also which protein foods are going to have the lowest and highest fat profile. Whereas the fat content of fat is pretty easy to measure, particularly if it comes in a bottle, tub, or stick, protein is somewhat more difficult. Protein energy foods contain only a portion of their calories from protein. How many calories come from fat in nuts, for example, is markedly different from that in meat.

As we shall discuss in the next section on fats, some fats are better than others, and for the most part, those we get from vegetable foods are more desirable, gram for gram, than those we get from animal foods. The exceptions are the omega-3 fatty acids derived from fatty fish. Tuna, mackerel, salmon, herring, anchovies, lake trout, shad and whitefish contain large amounts of omega-3 fatty acids, a type of healthy, polyunsaturated fat.

The following table lists the general kinds of protein energy foods available to us. None is pure protein.

percentages of protein in protein foods

Protein Energy Foods	% of calories from protein
meat and fish	30–50%
pulses (legumes)	20–36%
nuts and seeds	11–16%
cereals	8–16%
eggs	31%
milk*	21–39%
vegetables	10–33%

*This value is for whole milk. Other dairy products, such as cheeses and yogurt, will have differing values. Generally speaking, the drier the product, the higher its percentage of protein and particularly fat.

The following table lists common protein energy foods and their average fat component.

percentages of fat

Protein Food	Percentage of Calories from Fats
Nuts and seeds	73–95%
Meat (domesticated red meat)*	20–80%
Other meats (wild land animals)	Lower than domesticated meats, with a lower percentage of saturated fat
Cheese	13–90%
Eggs	65%
Cow's milk	50%
Poultry (water fowl higher than chicken and other land fowl)	8–56%
Fish	5–60%
Legumes	1.5–8%
Cereals (oats are highest; white rice lowest)	0.5–15%
Vegetables and fruits (except avocados and olives)	0–7%

*Try to limit red meat intake to no more than 10 percent of your daily energy supply. At an average 2000 calorie/day energy intake per day, this works out to a limit of about 3 ounces per day.

It is the AICR panel's recommendation that our dietary protein be derived mainly from vegetable, fish, poultry, and game, if possible, rather than from domesticated red meats. There are a number of good reasons for this. Fat is an important issue—the fats from animal sources tend to be largely saturated and will raise LDL (the bad cholesterol)—but research indicates, as noted above, that vegetable proteins are better for you. In addition to containing much lower levels of fats and very low levels of saturated fats, they are most often accompanied by valuable dietary fibers, phytochemicals, vitamins, minerals, and other dietary micronutrients that most animal proteins do not contain. Certainly meats are good sources of amino acids, vitamins, and minerals—red meat, for example, is a wonderful source of iron. But vegetable sources of protein, such as legumes and soy foods, are overall better for the planet as well: It takes considerably less waste, energy, and pollution, to produce a pound of lentils, than it does to produce a pound of beef.

fat and cholesterol

Fat is the most dense of our energy sources, with more than twice the calories by weight of carbohydrate or protein. It has been targeted over the last several years—and not without reason—as the chief evil of the American diet.

Despite its apparent dangers at inappropriate levels, fat is crucial to the metabolism of fat-soluble vitamins (A, D, E, K), crucial to the construction of cell membranes, and crucial to many other metabolic functions. It is also, at a certain point, the body's preferred source of energy. Fat is essential for survival, and it is particularly important in the diets of children younger than two years of age (and should not be restricted in babies up to two years). But like salt, iron, and any number of nutrients we cannot live without, a little bit goes a long way. Overabundance of dietary fat, particularly the wrong kinds of fat, can wreak all kinds of metabolic havoc, increasing your risk not only for cancer but for cardiovascular disease, diabetes, and many other chronic illnesses.

The good kinds of fats, in proper measure, can have numerous beneficial effects, so the overall goal in diet should be to get the right kinds of fats in the right proportions. The question then arises: How do we get to that goal?

If you've been wary of fat in your diet, looking for leaner meat and poultry, lower-fat foods and snacks, there's every reason to do so, even if there is still a considerable amount of confusion at large about what fats are good. Americans eat measurably less fat than they did even just a few years ago, yet Americans are also considerably heavier today than they were then. Rates of obesity, particularly among children, are rising at alarming rates. We will, in the following pages, try to clear up some of this seemingly contradictory information.

One of the problems with high fat diets is that they tend to be deficient in nutrient foods, ruling out the potential benefits of all those vitamins, minerals, phytochemicals, antioxidants, and other cancer-fighting bioactive compounds. High fat diets also tend to be characterized by empty calories (those from fats as well as those from simple sugars and starches) than lower fat diets.

And of course diets high in fats tend to be higher in calories, tend to put us in a positive energy balance, and increase the risk of obesity—all of which make the average, high-fat Western diet a factor in those many cancers whose risk is increased by obesity.

If you've been wary of fat in your diet, do you know why? Is it just because they're fats?

Some people have picked up the mistaken notion that calories are okay as long as they're not calories from fat—that simply by reducing intake of calories from fats, they're going to get fewer calories overall. There has arisen the myth that body fat and dietary fat are somehow the same—as long as something is low-fat, it won't makes us fat. *But this is most definitely not the case.*

Marketing geniuses have figured out that you can slap a "no-fat" label on a food, even a candy, and people will scoop them up like proverbial hotcakes, regardless of their calorie content. Those colorful, chewy little candy bears, made almost entirely of simple sugars—and almost pure calories—enjoyed only flat sales in this country for decades until someone slapped a fat-free label on them. What happened? Sales skyrocketed. No one, it is safe to say, is getting thin by eating candy, fat-free or not.

Compare the Nutrition Facts label on a box of no- or low-fat cookies with that on a package of conventional cookies. Ignoring the fat content for the moment, how do they compare in terms of total calories? Probably about the same; the low-fat version may have even more.

Regardless of its source, a calorie that isn't burned is going to turn to body fat (and this includes calories from alcohol). So even if you eat no-fat cookies and cakes and pies all night long, you're still going to develop body fat if you're not also out chopping wood, running, dancing, skating, sweating, and burning off all those calories. Desserts and sweets, fat-free or not, are going to have high levels of calories—mostly empty calories.

The whole point of sweet indulgences is sweet indulgence, which, everything in balance, is more or less a fine treat once in a while. But don't harbor any illusions that as long as it's fat-free, you can eat as much as you want and you're not going to get fat.

That said, it makes sense to look into fats, what they are, what they do, and what they mean in your diet—and how much of a place they should hold.

the butter vs. margarine debate

There's a naked baked potato sitting on your dinner plate. Which is a healthier topping for that steaming spud—a pat of butter or margarine? The correct answer, until recently, was thought to be margarine. Now health experts say it's not so simple.

Several years ago, the nation's health officials recommended replacing butter with margarine whenever possible. Although both contain an equal number of calories and fat grams (one hundred calories and eleven grams of fat in a tablespoon), butter is higher in saturated fat—about eight grams of saturated fat to margarine's two grams per tablespoon. Cutting your consumption of saturated fat may lower your blood cholesterol level and reduce your risk for heart disease. Butter also contains cholesterol, which margarine does not.

Enter trans-fatty acids, the new villains on the fat scene that have sullied margarine's image. Trans-fatty acids are the result of hydrogenation, or the artificial saturation of fat. Margarine, vegetable shortening and the partially-hydrogenated oils used to make cookies, crackers and other such products all contain trans-fatty acids.

Many health experts feel that too little is known about the effects of trans-fatty acids on the body to reverse the earlier recommendations. Health-conscious consumers who have made the switch from butter to margarine feel understandably frustrated by the conflicting information. What to do?

It's important to note that trans-fats exist in nature at relatively low levels, and have only been a significant part of human diet for about the last forty to seventy years. Their highest concentration is actually not in margarine, but in processed foods: the hydrogenated shortenings used to make foods such as cookies, french fries, crackers, and donuts.

It's also worth noting that not all margarines are the same when it comes to trans-fats. Soft, tub margarines are significantly lower in trans-fatty acids than harder stick margarines. Some soft, reduced-fat margarine spreads have more water and less fat, including less trans-fats, although most of these reduced-fat spreads are not suitable for baking.

AICR believes the important point is not which is better, but that butter, margarine and all other types of fat should be consumed only in moderation. Instead of butter or margarine on your baked potato, there are lots of different ways you can flavor it without even using fat. A lot of people use reduced-fat or fat-free yogurt in place of sour cream. Add a little of that, your favorite herbs, some salsa, nonfat sour cream, nonfat cottage cheese—the alternatives are only as limited as your imagination—and you can have a tasty baked potato, leaving out the fat completely.

A diet low in total fat—both saturated and unsaturated—can lower your risk for cancers of the colon, prostate, and breast. If your overall diet is low in fat, if you're in good energy balance and exercising regularly, an occasional pat of butter or margarine is not a problem.

what is fat?

In the same way that protein and carbohydrate are not just protein or carbohydrate but building blocks, so it is with fat. In the case of fat, the building blocks are what is known as *fatty acids,* or chains of carbon atoms with hydrogen atoms attached. The chains are capped off by a carbon atom attached to two molecules of oxygen, known as a *carboxyl acid group.*

Nearly all the fat we eat (more than 90 percent) comes in the form of *triglycerides* (also known as triacylglycerols), which are three chains of fatty acids bonded to a glycerol (alcohol) molecule. Chains of fatty acids come in varying lengths and in differing levels of saturation. When we eat fat, it's digested in the small intestine, and a healthy small intestine will absorb nearly every bit of fat we eat.

Fats are not water soluble, but are somewhat soluble in alcohol. Since they're not water-soluble, the process by which they are broken down and reassembled into usable energy is somewhat more involved than the digestion of proteins and carbohydrates.

Bile, produced by the liver and stored in the gall bladder, is released when we eat. It acts as a detergent to help split the large droplets of triglycerides into smaller droplets, making them more easily broken down by digestive enzymes. This is the same way laundry detergent will break down grease stains on your clothing. Laundry detergent and digestive enzymes are actually made from similar compounds.

These digestive enzymes, known as *lipases,* are produced by the pancreas and break triglycerides down into their building blocks—individual fatty acids, monoglycerides (also known as monoacylglycerols), and glycerol.

Once absorbed, short- and medium-chain fatty acids are transported to the liver in the blood. Long-chain fatty acids and cholesterol (which is not a fat, but is made from fats and is also insoluble in water), are reassembled in the intestinal wall into lipoproteins. These then flow through the lymphatic system, and eventually join the bloodstream. As lipoproteins move through the body, many give up their triglycerides to fat cells and muscles along the way. Fats and cholesterol remaining in the bloodstream pass through the liver, where they are reorganized into various lipoproteins. These are eventually returned to the bloodstream, where, as before, they deliver their components to various tissues.

If you've ever heard that fats are "hard to digest," this multistage approach to the breakdown and reassembly of fats in the digestive tract may help explain why.

Fat, of course, is energy and can be burned as energy. If the tissues that pick up fats as they're transported through your bloodstream happen to be muscles or other lean body tissues that are working, the fats will likely be burned. When you exercise, carbohydrate tends to be burned first, because it's most readily available. But available carbohydrate is depleted relatively rapidly, and after about twenty minutes or so of exercise, depending upon its intensity, your tissues start burning fat. But if those lean body tissues happen not to need any energy, the leftover fats are going to go straight into storage as body fat.

A certain amount of this is healthy. It's good and natural to maintain a certain level of body fat: It helps retain body heat, provides us with an all-important store of energy, and offers protection for the skin and organs. In addition it helps us retain moisture, and our cells are made up in part from it. But you don't want to keep enough body fat hanging around to warm the whole house. The accumulation of body fat beyond the ideal point makes for a vicious cycle. It provokes insulin resistance, which has been linked to cancers, as well as to cardiovascular disease and diabetes mellitus. Insulin, as noted previously, is an anabolic steroid, or tissue-building hormone. It can help build lean body tissue, but if you become insulin resistant, it mainly builds more fat, which is where the vicious cycle comes in. The higher your ratio of fat to lean body mass, the more fat you're going to create because you're going to have more triglycerides in your bloodstream at any given time, and high triglycerides have been shown to create insulin-resistance. When you become insulin-resistant, your body makes more insulin, and it goes out and does its job, which is create fat.

essential fatty acids

As we've stated, a little bit of fat goes a long way. Most of the fats the body needs can be manufactured from other dietary macronutrients. Still, there are fatty acids that are essential. One essential fatty acid (EFA) is linoleic acid. This is a polyunsaturated, omega-6 fatty acid that can be had from a number of plant sources, such as vegetable oils, and also from animal sources such as fish oils, mean, and milk. The other EFA is alpha-*linolenic acid,* a polyunsaturated omega-3 fatty acid. It can be found in fish and canola oil, as well as in leafy green vegetables, nuts, seeds, and soybeans. Linoleic, arachidonic, eicosopentanoic,[27] and related fatty acids are precursors to prostaglandins, which are hormone-like compounds that perform a number of different functions in the metabolic process, including roles in blood vessel dilation/constriction, blood clotting, the control of inflammation, and the transmission of nerve impulses. The balance of fats in the system is also quite important, because overloading with one kind of fat can lead to the production of unneeded fatty acids and underproduction of needed fatty acids.

Dutch researchers Bang and Dyerberg conducted studies of Eskimos, who derive a high percentage of their dietary energy from fat (mainly from

---

[27] These Greek-rooted names for fatty acids are derived from the numbers of fatty acids in their chains.

fatty, cold water fish), yet have a low incidence of cardiovascular disease and obesity. These surprising findings sparked further research into the omega-3 fatty acids, especially eicospentanoic acid (EPA)—and probably are the root of the recent industry in fish oil supplements. Although EPA can be synthesized from alpha-linolenic acid in humans, it is by no means guaranteed. This is because the enzymatic processes by which one fatty acid is converted to another have their limitations, and dietary fats tend to compete for those enzymes. So this synthesis can be slow or even nonexistent if dietary levels of the omega-6 fatty acids linoleic (an EFA) and arachidonic acid are high. What happens is that these fatty acids get converted to other, perhaps less beneficial fatty acids. The best source of EPA is fish, which gets this cancer-protective and heart-healthy fatty acid directly into your system so the competition needn't take place. This is why one of AICR's recommendations is to work fish into your diet at least twice a week. Don't fry it, which will add other fats—bake or poach it. Or if you do cook it with added fat, use a little olive oil.

saturation

No doubt you've heard of saturated, polyunsaturated, and monounsaturated fats, and perhaps even of trans-fatty acids, but what does saturation tell us about fat? Does saturated fat have more calories than unsaturated fat?[28] Is saturated fat worse for you than unsaturated fat? Is saturated fat the "good" fat and unsaturated the "bad"? Or vice versa? And does whether you eat saturated fat or unsaturated fat increase your risk of cancer?

In all fats, each of the roughly two to twenty carbon atoms in a fatty acid chain is bonded together. *Saturation* refers to the amount of hydrogen that saturates the bond. If a bond holds as much hydrogen as it can, it's known as saturated.

In meat, butter, lard, and coconut oil, approximately 45 to 50 percent of the fat is saturated. The fat in poultry and eggs is roughly 25 to 30 percent saturated (most of the fat in eggs is in the yolks). In vegetable oils, about 6 to 20 percent of the fat is saturated; in soft margarines, about 17 percent. The fat in fish is approximately 10 to 35 percent saturated.

---

[28] The answer to this question is no, saturated fat has the same number of calories per gram as the unsaturated fats.

Saturated fats (and trans-fatty acids, which are unsaturated fats that have had extra hydrogen added in order to make them more stable) tend to be the fats of choice for food manufacturers because of their stability. Since there is no place for an oxygen molecule to attach, they do not oxidize (or turn rancid) as rapidly as unsaturated fats, and therefore have a longer shelf life. If oxidation can be harmful, then why aren't saturated fats better fats that unsaturated?

Dietary saturated fat comes mostly from animal foods, and as such it also tends to be accompanied by dietary cholesterol (which only comes from animal foods). Saturated fat has the unpleasant effect of raising LDL (the bad cholesterol). So when eating animal fats, your body may not only acquire extra cholesterol, it will likely manufacture more of its own bad cholesterol. Does this mean that saturated fat is necessarily bad? No, not necessarily. Particularly not if you're burning if as you eat it.

But if you're not burning it, and many of us aren't, that's another story. In a sense, this stability of saturated fat may be nature's design—if it lasts longer on the shelf without oxidizing, it may be nature's storage form of fat. It's interesting to note that some of the most common saturated fats are used to make things like candles and wood finishes.

Saturated fats tend to be quite orderly in shape, so they nestle very nicely together and form solids at room temperature. Pretty much any fat that's solid at room temperature is going to be predominantly saturated.

Trans-fat is a fat that begins life as an unsaturated fatty acid. It becomes more saturated by adding heat and hydrogen (when you see "partially hydrogenated vegetable oil" on an ingredients list, it means the food contains trans-fat). *Trans* refers to the shape of the carbon chain. Most fats are "bent" in one direction. Fats that have been hydrogenated bend in the other direction, hence the designation *trans*. There is considerable debate over how good or bad for you trans-fatty acids may be. Trans-fatty acids came to public attention in May of 1994, when an article in the *American Journal of Public Health* stated that they may be worse than saturated fat. Like saturated fat, trans-fatty acids have been shown to increase the LDL cholesterol in your blood, though at only about half the amount as saturated fat. However, unlike saturated fat, they also may decrease the level of HDL (the good) cholesterol in your blood. Some researchers worry that since trans-fat in processed foods has only been around for about a century, the body may have no good means for utilizing or metabolizing large amounts of it, and it may therefore be more hazardous to human health than naturally saturated fats.

A monounsaturated fat in the carbon chain is not completely loaded with hydrogen. Monounsaturated fat tends to be more stable than polyunsaturated fat, which has two or more spots in the carbon chain not fully loaded (or "saturated") with hydrogen, and it doesn't break down as readily into oxidizable (and therefore potentially mutagenic) compounds, such as lipid peroxides, when it is heated. Monounsaturated fats are recommended for cooking. Also, monounsaturated fat does not raise LDL cholesterol or lower HDL (good) cholesterol. The predominant monounsaturated fatty acid is oleic acid, which has its richest source in olives. The oils of choice for cooking and salad dressings and so on should be olive oil or canola, another primarily monounsaturated fat.

does fat increase cancer risk?

There is a consistent pattern of research evidence to suggest that diets high in total fat may increase the risk of lung, colorectal, breast, and prostate cancers; and that diets high in animal fat (largely saturated fat) may increase the risk of lung, colorectal, breast, and prostate cancers. And there is evidence that diets high in dietary cholesterol[29] seem to lead to an increase in the risk of lung and pancreatic cancers.

The evidence that obesity increases the risk of endometrial cancer is convincing. Obesity has also been linked to an increase in the risk of postmenopausal breast and renal (kidney) cancers.

Fat has been studied extensively in the context of those cancers that are more common in the developed world, including those associated with obesity. A National Academy of Sciences report concluded that, of all the dietary components it reviewed, the evidence for a causal relationship between dietary fat and cancer was strongest, particularly for cancers of the breast and colon. One of that report's six dietary guidelines recommended reduction of total fat intake to 30 percent total energy, adding "the

---

[29] Dietary cholesterol is that which is eaten and its sole dietary source is animal foods. It is not an essential nutrient—the body manufactures its own—and you can get along fine without dietary cholesterol. It is similar in structure to bile acids, sex hormones, adrenal hormones, and vitamin D, and is an important precursor (raw material) in their production by the body, although in what has become the Western/developed world diet it too often falls into the "too much of a good thing" category.

scientific data do not provide a strong basis for establishing fat intake at precisely 30 percent total calories. Indeed, the data could be used to justify an even greater reduction."

The Surgeon General's 1988 report *Nutrition and Health,* and the NAS's 1989 report both recommended a reduction in intakes of total and saturated fat and cholesterol. The NAS report concluded that the weight of evidence supported a relationship between high-fat diets and cancers of the colon, prostate, and breast. The World Health Organization's 1990 report, *Diet, Nutrition and the Prevention of Chronic Diseases,* also concluded that diets containing large amounts of total fat were associated with an increased risk of cancers of the colon, prostate and breast, and that obesity was associated with endometrial cancer.

The answer, as you may already have guessed, is that it seems likely that the intake of excess dietary fat does indeed increase cancer risk, although the mechanisms by which it may increase risk are yet a little murky. There is, however, no question that a high-calorie, positive energy-balance diet that leads to obesity will increase your risk of cancer.

the take-home message on fats and cancer

It bears repeating that a little bit of fat goes a long way. All of the essential fatty acids your body needs can be had from a balanced diet and about a teaspoon a day of almost any vegetable oil. Given what most of us eat, that's a lot of fat that can go by the wayside.

But it should be remembered that the omega-3 fats do seem to be beneficial in many ways. Their best source is fatty, cold water fish, so try to include fish regularly in your diet. Try to limit meats and saturated fats as much as possible. And while research suggests that there is no reason to avoid adding monounsaturated oils to food, it should be done so that the total fat in the diet stays within recommended limits.

alcohol

There has been a fair amount of media coverage of the so-called French paradox, or the apparent ability of the French to smoke like Humphrey Bogart, eat a diet loaded with fats, and still have lower rates of obesity, heart disease, and cancer overall than supposedly health-conscious Americans. Often cited as an underlying reason for the French paradox is the French consumption of red wine—and the French have one of the highest rates of consumption of alcohol in the world. The tannins and bioactive chemicals that make the wine red are often credited for why red wine may be "healthy" for the French. White wine, it is said, does not have a similar effect.

A recent study conducted by the French government showed, however, that the French paradox is largely mythical. That study broke France into regions and compared the death rates of the various regions by cause, and also compared life expectancy. Those who lived near the German border had a life expectancy (and lifestyle/diet) much like the Germans—the shortest life expectancy in France. It is in those regions where most of the smoking, drinking and fatty-food eating takes place. In the Mediterranean region, where the consumption of fresh vegetables and fruits is highest, so is the life expectancy. Toulouse, which has the highest consumption of tomatoes per capita in France, had the longest life expectancy—close to a decade more than some other regions.

Wine and alcohol in general consumed in small quantities may have some beneficial effects on health (red wine does seem to lower LDL cholesterol somewhat, and have other not-entirely-understood heart-health benefits). Alcohol, however, has no established protective effect at all for cancer. Quite the opposite: Alcoholic drinks have such a profound effect on increased risk of cancer that it has been classified since 1988 by the International Agency for Research on Cancer (IARC) as a class 1 carcinogen for cancers of the liver and much of the upper aerodigestive tract: mouth, pharynx, larynx, and esophagus. (A class 1 carcinogen is the top rating of how likely a substance is to be carcinogenic in humans.)

Although the body uses alcohols in different ways, there is no dietary need for it whatsoever. There are populations that, mainly for religious reasons, avoid alcohol entirely, and their cancer rates, as well as health in general, is much better than that of other populations that do drink. (Certainly the argument can be made that these populations also make lots of other "clean" lifestyle choices because of their religious beliefs. But if alcohol acts as a powerful promoter of cancer, that would only seem to bolster the argument that alcohol, in combination with other lifestyle factors, only increases the likelihood of cancer.)

While ethanol (the form of alcohol found in alcoholic beverages, regardless of whether the drink is wine, beer, or spirits) is a more concentrated source of calories than either carbohydrate or protein (nearly twice as many, by weight), it shouldn't amount to a significant portion of *anyone's* daily caloric intake.[30] When it does amount to a significant proportion of caloric intake, if the individual is in energy balance, that would indicate a significant loss elsewhere in the diet. Studies have shown that most often, in the case of people who drink regularly, this is the case.

Studies have also shown that smoking and drinking go hand in hand. Smokers, on average, are much more likely to be regular drinkers than nonsmokers. Nearly every study of the nutritional intake of smokers (and of the blood concentrations of important nutrients—for example, vitamin C) have shown that smokers usually have poorer overall nutrition than nonsmokers (nicotine having well-known appetite-suppressant qualities), sometimes considerably so. In both drinkers and smokers, the loss to the diet tends to be just the foods that might help them the most—vegetables and fruits. There are aspects of such studies that show that smokers may actually need more of these important nutrient foods than nonsmokers because smoking appears to impede the ability to metabolize many important nutrients.

does alcohol increase cancer risk?

There's no way to avoid the facts: yes.

Alcohol has been linked to cancer since the last century when it was noted that many patients with cancers of the esophagus were alcoholics or worked in the alcohol trade.

Expert reports on diet and cancer generally specify alcohol as a risk factor for cancers of various sites when alcohol is counted as part of diet. Groundbreaking researchers Doll and Peto concluded in 1981 that alcohol accounted for 3 percent of cancer deaths in the United States, adding that "the totality of the evidence suggests that the principal effect is due to the alcohol itself and is largely independent of the form in which it is drunk."

---

[30] At about 200 calories per ounce of pure alcohol, that amount (which would be about two glasses of wine, two bottles of beer, or two mixed drinks) would be 10 percent of our average 2000 calorie daily intake. Any given drink can, however, contain significant numbers of additional calories from carbohydrate, particularly in beer or mixed drinks, usually in the form of fast-acting sugars and starches. Certain chemicals in dark beer have been linked to a higher cancer risk.

However, given the synergistic effect on upper aerodigestive cancers of smoking with drinking, they further stated: "Most of the three percent of cancer deaths now caused by alcohol could have been avoided by the absence of smoking, even if alcohol consumption remained unchanged."

The NAS recommended in 1982 that "if alcoholic beverages be consumed, it be done in moderation," having reviewed the evidence then available on alcohol and cancers of the upper aerodigestive tract (synergistic with smoking), colorectal cancer (mentioning a possible link between beer and rectal cancer) and liver cancer (as a consequence of cirrhosis).

In 1988, as noted above, the IARC concluded that there was "suggestive but inconclusive" evidence of a causal link with cancer of the rectum. On breast cancer the report concluded that "the modest elevation in relative risk that has been observed is potentially important because of the high incidence of breast cancer in many countries. Although the available data indicate a positive association between drinking of alcoholic beverages and breast cancer in women, a firm conclusion about a causal relationship cannot be made at present."

The report also concluded that there was little or no indication that the effects of alcohol on the risk of cancer of any site were dependent upon the type of drink. The 1989 NAS report concluded, after reviewing the evidence on alcohol and cancer as well as other diseases, that "the committee does not recommend alcohol consumption," and proposed an upper limit of less than 1 ounce (28 grams) of pure alcohol a day.

the take-home message on alcohol and cancer

The finding of the AICR expert panel was that for the lowest possible cancer risk, alcohol should be avoided. If you do drink, limit consumption as much as possible. For women, this means an *upper* limit of one drink per day; for men, an *upper* limit of two drinks per day. (A drink is defined as 1½ ounces of distilled 80-proof liquor, 12 ounces of beer, or 5 ounces of wine.) These recommendations are one of the few cases in this book when we are *not* talking about averages. This doesn't mean you should save up your drinks for a Saturday night binge. While a single binge of six or seven drinks—say, on New Year's Eve—may not increase your risk of cancer, but common sense says it very well may.

9

nutrient foods

When we talk about nutrient foods, we are mainly talking about those foods we turn to for their vitamins, minerals, and of course their flavor, rather than for their energy. For most of us, while we may not necessarily be deficient in our RDAs, this group of foods is probably where our diets go wanting. When things get hectic, there just aren't that many drive-up windows where you can get a spinach and broccoli salad with a glass of tomato juice on the side. And so the foods we grab all tend to be from the energy category—burgers and fries, chips, nuts, donuts, and so on. Most of our lives are hectic, and while it's the nutrient foods that would help us stay fitter and healthier and quicker on our feet (not to mention better equipped to avoid cancer), it's the nutrient foods, statistically, that we tend to miss out on the most.

Vegetables and fruits make up the largest portion of our nutrient foods, but these are by no means the only ones. In fact, many of the foods that fall into this category we may not think of as foods at all. Herbs, spices, and other flavorings are examples. You wouldn't exactly think of having a plate of oregano or sage or rosemary for lunch, or for that matter, a few cloves of garlic, but you'd certainly think of adding them to your cooking. And depending upon what you're making, these little health-promoting power-houses may just be the most cancer-preventive part of your meal. So nutrient foods, as we're categorizing them, contain in addition to vegetables and fruits other foods of plant origin—herbs, spices, and any other food or fla-voring we might eat that comes from plant sources.

Nutrients are conventionally understood as macronutrients (the energy foods) and micronutrients—vitamins, minerals, and so on. But nutrient foods contain many "unconventional nutrients." These compounds have considerable bioactive cancer-fighting potential, and, although in a less well-understood way, may be as important to health as conventionally understood nutrients. These chemicals, referred to here under the broad category of *bioactive compounds,* have—thanks to scientific advances over the last two decades—only recently begun to be understood.

Researchers have begun to discover that vitamins and minerals long understood to be essential nutrients have considerably more value than simply preventing diseases of deficiency. Indeed, in the common vegetables and fruits we eat, as well as in the herbs and spices, there are uncounted thousands of nutrient compounds. Working synergistically with the vita-mins and minerals that accompany them, these nutrients are being shown to go a long way toward protecting us against cancer. But unlike the energy foods, they seem to have almost no roll in at all of promoting any kind of cancer.

As discussed previously, much of conventional nutritional advice and much of the mindset of conventional nutritional thinking has, over this cen-tury, been occupied by the very sensible and useful goal of preventing nutritional deficiency. (This is not to diminish or discount the importance of not being deficient—diseases of deficiency can have truly horrible con-sequences.) Nutritional deficiency is no longer the central health concern of most Americans. Indeed, over the last twenty years or so, the central health concern of most Americans has shifted to chronic illness—cancer, cardiovascular disease, diabetes, obesity and related diseases. Many if not most chronic illnesses can be reversed, improved, or prevented outright by dietary changes that emphasize these nutrient foods.

There are, however, initiatives to make the public more aware of the health value of nutrient foods. The National Cancer Institute, for example, encourages people to eat five or more servings of vegetables and fruits a day.[31]

Which again brings up the important question: What is a serving of fruits and vegetables, anyway?

A serving of fruits and vegetables is pretty much what seems like a serving. A peach. A bunch of grapes. A couple of serving spoons of sautéed zucchini or steamed stringbeans. A bowl of berries.

A considerable amount of research into diet since the 1980s has shown that consuming nutrient foods at rates far higher than any recommended minimums can have considerable health benefits.

At least twenty studies have been performed on rodents in which cancer was deliberately induced with chemical or other carcinogens. In the vast majority of these trials, researchers found that the animals that were fed vegetables or fruits experienced fewer and smaller tumors, fewer metastases (tumors spreading to other sites), less DNA damage, and higher levels of the enzymes involved with the detoxification of the carcinogens. In most of the studies, the proportionate amounts of the vegetables included in the animals' diets were, relatively speaking, well above those amounts typically eaten by humans. And all the evidence indicates that the higher the intake, the lower the risk.

There is, of course, always some difficulty in translating the results of animal experiments to humans, but there have also been numerous studies of humans (some of which we will discuss at greater length later) that link a lower incidence of cancer of nearly every variety with diets higher in vegetables and fruits. This is true even of smokers: those with a higher vegetable and fruit intake also show a lower likelihood of getting cancer. If they stopped smoking entirely, their risk would plummet.

Diets high in nutrient foods don't just help protect against cancer. There is substantial evidence that diets high in vegetables and fruits protect against a number of other chronic diseases. For example, diets high in foods rich in carotenoids, vitamin C, and possibly other antioxidants, protect against cataracts. They also decrease the oxidation of cholesterol in the arteries and thus protect against cardiovascular disease. Vitamin C may

---

[31] The number five is a minimum figure, adopted as a compromise. More servings would be even better, but the NCI's scientists feared that too high a figure would scare people away from vegetables and fruits completely.

help maximize intestinal iron absorption and thereby help prevent anemia.

Many vegetables and fruits are high in NSP fiber, and in potassium. NSP fiber may help control diabetes and high serum cholesterol levels, and it most certainly protects against diverticular disease and many other digestive disorders. Potassium, present at some level in nearly all vegetables and fruits, is crucial to cellular function and may help prevent or control hypertension, thereby reducing the subsequent risk of stroke and heart disease. It may also work in tandem with other minerals to keep the cells functioning at optimum levels, which means better overall health and disease-fighting ability.

But this notion of the beneficial effects of very high intakes of vegetables and fruits is really quite new. The concept that some other microconstituents (micronutrients) of diet (many of which, such as antioxidants, few of us had heard of twenty years ago) may be protective against chronic disease, even in the absence of any known or presently definable state of deficiency, is even more recent. This means that in many respects, for optimum health, and optimum cancer protection, we must radically rethink our attitudes toward nutrient foods. It also means that most of us should radically alter the amounts of these foods in our diets.

If the nutrient foods are so good for us, so marvelously healthy, why don't we eat more of them? Why do we Americans eat only about three-quarters of the minimum the government recommends we should?

It's a good question, and one that probably has many different answers. It may have to do with misunderstanding the value of nutrient foods and the relative risks and benefits of energy foods.

For many of us with breakneck lifestyles, there is the question of convenience. A banana may be convenient to throw in your purse or your briefcase for a snack, and so may many other fruits—oranges, apples, pears—but many nutrient foods require at least a little preparation. Celery stalks need to be washed and cut; carrots need to be peeled (although you can now buy bags of cut and shaped and washed carrots that make a fine snack). And nearly everything requires washing. If you can snack on a bag of chips or grab a burger in the drive-through, why bother with the fruits and veggies? At least you can get everything you need from a vitamin supplement. *Wrong!*

And there's the question of freshness: Fruits and vegetables have their highest nutrient value if harvested at peak ripeness and eaten within about three days. This is often not possible, given the logistics of getting fruits and vegetables to market. Which is fresher, strawberries frozen shortly after picking, or "fresh" strawberries that have been on a truck for a day or more, and then on your grocer's shelf for two or three days, and then perhaps in your refrigerator for a day or two? How about stringbeans that have been canned or frozen right at harvest, or stringbeans that have been on a truck, then your grocer's shelf, then your refrigerator?

If you want fresh fruits and vegetables, again, the convenience question comes up: you have to shop for them every three or four days or they lose flavor and begin to rot (but you're supposed to *eat* them, remember, not let them sit). Don't think of frozen or canned vegetables as not fresh (but do look out for added salts and sugars). Frozen or canned fruits and vegetables can be a very sensible alternative.

contaminants, chemicals, & additives

Contaminants, chemicals, and additives worry a lot of people. The belief that particular additives or contaminants are a significant cause of cancer is typical of the general misunderstanding of how cancer happens and the mistaken notion that cancer is mostly caused by exposure to single carcinogens. Media coverage of cancer research often unintentionally reinforces this idea, particularly when it tries to promote a "balanced" view of the news. Single agents can cause cancer (and in research in lab animals, cancer is deliberately induced by single, known carcinogenic agents). But as discussed earlier, only a very small percentage of cancers happens this way in humans.

There is no doubt that food and drink can occasionally be contaminated. Many powerful chemicals are used in modern agri-business. However, a powerful chemical in the field or at the factory does not necessarily translate to a powerful chemical at your table. Still, there are chemicals that are worrisome. Over the years the use and disposal of industrial chemicals has been subject to increasingly stringent regulation. However, problems remain. While we cannot be complacent about the presence in food of chemicals known to be mutagenic or carcinogenic, we must also be realistic. Substances known to be toxic to laboratory animals may have no effect on humans. The reverse may also be true. Safety evaluations often are based on untested assumptions.

Also, chemicals may interact with each other and become more or less toxic in tandem than alone, although clear evidence for this is not available.

The exact implications for the risk of cancer or other diseases as a result of exposure to chemical or other contamination in general are not clear. Any judgments made on the safety of chemical residues are based on regulations issued by international and national bodies. We cannot necessarily apply these to parts of the world that do not recognize such regulations, or in cases of abuse, spillage or accidents.

Expert reports assessing the role of chemical residues in human cancer risk—compared with those assessing the risk of diets as a whole—have generally come to the view that residues are relatively unimportant factors. You may worry if you ish to about the strange chemical names on the ingredients label of your food, but from a health perspective the sugars and fats may do you much more harm. Nonetheless, we cannot say unequivocally that chemical residues are unimportant.

The pesticide DDT, for example, which can take much of the credit for the demise of malaria in this country, is unfortunately poisonous to humans as well as mosquitoes. Although it has been banned in this country for many years, it takes a very long time to decompose, and residues of it are still present in the soil throughout the country. It is still in use in other countries, so traces can show up in both domestic and imported foods and drinks. But even research on DDT residues is as yet inconclusive as to whether it is responsible for an increase in cancer risk.

Foods and drinks can also be contaminated by the use of chemical additives. Packaged foods might be contaminated by chemicals in plastics. Food and drink can also be contaminated by flawed processing and handling. This kind of contamination leads to more of a risk of bacterial infection than increasing cancer risk, but some kinds of contamination (as with certain molds) have been shown to increase cancer risk.

Figuring out exactly what effect residues in food can have is difficult: On-the-job overexposure can be hazardous, and environmental pollution caused by improper use—as with pesticide spray drift or by industrial accidents, such as those in Seveso and Bhopal—can be outright deadly or can markedly increase cancer risk. But used in the way they are intended, such chemicals should pose—and indeed the statistics indicate that they do pose—little risk for the general population.

the take-home message on contaminants, additives, and residues

Public wariness of chemicals in foods is understandable but disproportionate to the cancers actually caused by such chemicals. Used in agriculture and food processing as intended, most chemicals are safe and not a significant cause of cancer. Because some chemical residues are known to accumulate in fat-containing foods (particularly in animal fat), this is yet another reason to try to reduce your intake of fats, particularly saturated fats. While concentrations of contaminants in fish and seafood as a result of dumping in rivers and seas can in some cases be quite high, most fish is quite safe and a desirable part of the diet.

But the unfortunate fact is that many of us have probably had some pretty miserable culinary experiences with vegetables—for instance, in a cafeteria line: overcooked, oversalted vegetables gleaming with some fatty, unidentifiable butter-substitute, all the nutrition and flavor leached out of them from hours of boiling. How many of us haven't had peas and stringbeans and even Brussels sprouts that, instead of popping on your tongue with sugary freshness as they should, glob on your plate with the consistency of toothpaste?

Or fruits: Apples that should pop when your teeth break the skin instead turn into mealy mush; peaches that should bleed sweet nectar down your arm when you bite into them, instead have the consistency of wet sawdust.

But to avoid vegetables and fruits for these reasons is to invite cancer. To think you're going to get all the nutrients your body needs by using supplement tablets or capsules is to fool yourself. Even worse, it's to miss out on some of the best-tasting foods available. You could take antioxidants as dietary supplements along with your vitamin pill, but you still won't even approach the true health value of a diet very high in vegetables and fruits. (It's been shown in various studies, as we shall discuss, that the quasi-pharmacological approach to using antioxidants—taking them as pills—doesn't do much good, and in some cases may do harm. There are so many cancer-fighting compounds working together in these foods that separating them from one another in supplements appears to have very little benefit. And why bother? They'd be exponentially more expensive.) The point is also that none of us should miss out on all the really good tastes that fresh herbs, vegetables, fruits, and a little fresh knowledge can bring.

Whether they're canned, frozen, or fresh, nutrient foods don't have to be a hassle. These foods are more than worth every moment of preparation time. When preparing your fruits and vegetables (if not eating them raw, which is certainly easiest), you can be as creative as you want to be (and we're perfectly willing to help out on that score; see Recipes), but the research shows that you will be rewarded in manifold ways.

the fresh food quandary

Do you avoid buying fresh vegetables because you think they'll spoil in your refrigerator before you can use them? There are a number of different ways you can improve the longevity of fresh vegetables and fruits in your home. Before you cross them off your shopping list, try these suggestions and see if they work for you:

- Shop with a friend. Try sharing a head of dark green, leafy lettuce or bunch of celery. (Eat with friends, too. If you're single, it's often much easier to prepare good food for two or three or four than just one, and more fun).
- Wash vegetables when ready to use—wet vegetables rot faster. Bunches of greens and heads of lettuce, however, can be washed all at once. Store the remaining greens in a plastic bag. The drier you can get them after washing it, the longer they will keep. Salad spinners are great for this, but don't pack them or they won't get dry. After your greens are spun, you can put a couple folded paper towels in the bag along with them to absorb excess water.
- Buy fruits and vegetables in season—they'll be cheaper, will more likely be from local sources, and this is really the way nature intended it. If you really take advantage of seasonal produce, by the time tomatoes and peppers are out of season, you'll be sick of them (but healthier for it), and ready to go onto the different delights of artichokes and spinach and chard and apples and fennel and squash and pumpkins, or whatever is in season.
- Pop unused portions of red and green peppers, fresh herbs, and other cleaned vegetables into a freezer bag to use in casseroles and other cooked dishes. (The broccoli you cooked but couldn't eat last night may go perfectly in Sunday evening's casserole.) You can do the same with berries—frozen strawberries, blueberries, blackberries, and so on go great in a fruit smoothie in the blender, mixed with fruit juice. Believe it or not, tofu can be a great thickener that's also good for you. Frozen fruits can also be turned into sorbet or other kinds of fruity, nutritious, cancer-fighting desserts.

- If you're too busy to peel and chop, buy small portions of fresh chopped vegetables from the grocery store salad bar. Some vitamins may be lost due to the slicing in advance, and there's the chance they might be a bit more expensive, but these are still a nutritious choice. Which is really more expensive, vegetables and fruits you eat, or the rotted ones you pitch?
- Choose fresh vegetables that keep well for a week or more: artichokes, beets, cabbage, carrots, celery, parsnips, pumpkins, onions, and radishes.
- Fruit that doesn't need to be refrigerated should be kept on the table where you will see it and be reminded to eat it. Remember, out-of-sight is often out-of-mind, so store refrigerated fruit in a bowl rather than in the crisper.
- Fresh produce is great, but don't be afraid to shop for frozen vegetables. They are about equal in nutritional value to truly fresh vegetables (but can actually be more nutritious than fresh vegetables shipped long distances) and they retain flavor and texture when microwaved, steamed, or marinated in a low-oil dressing for a myriad of different kinds of salads.

vegetables and fruits

There are several different kinds of fruits and vegetables. Each class or category has a different nutritional profile, and each has its own powerhouse of cancer-fighting properties. Since most of us should be getting many important nutrients from vegetables, let's talk about them first.

vegetables

Vegetables are, botanically speaking, any part of a plant not involved in the sexual reproduction of the plant, meaning that they are most often the leaves, roots, stalks, bulbs, and flowers. Some of the foods we normally call vegetables, such as tomatoes, cucumbers, peppers, squashes, and eggplant, are actually fruits, but the distinction isn't really that important. True vegetables include artichokes, asparagus, beets, broccoli, Brussels sprouts, cabbage, carrots, cauliflower, chard, endive, fennel, garlic, kohlrabi, leeks, lettuce, mushrooms, onions, parsley, parsnips, radishes, rhubarb, rutabaga, spinach, and turnips. Some of these, you'll notice, are the bulbs (garlic, onions, fennel), some the leaves (chard, spinach, endive), and some the stalks (broccoli, asparagus). But when we divide up the vegetables into their categories, as with the energy foods, we're not so much worried about the origin as we are about the kinds of nutrients they contain and how they work. Most of them have particular nutrients in common: green vegetables contain folates and vitamin C, for example, but have considerably different amounts of other vitamins, and different varieties of cancer-fighting compounds than, say, red and orange fruits and vegetables, such as carrots, tomatoes, peppers, berries, which are high in antioxidants, also have vitamin C, and are loaded with carotenoids. The most important thing to remember, in any case, is that the best, most cancer-healthy, diet is going to contain, on average, lots of different kinds of nutrient foods. Still, it can be helpful to know which classes of nutrient foods are the best sources of different biochemical goodies.

With that in mind, we can divide vegetables into the main categories of:

- **green leafy:** spinach, arugula, chard, lettuces, parsley, kale, collard greens
- **cruciferous:** broccoli, cauliflower, kohlrabi, Brussels sprouts, cabbage
- **allium:** onions, garlic, scallions, chives, shallots, leeks
- **non-starchy roots:** carrots, beets, turnips, and radishes, which are all technically tubers or roots, but classified here as vegetables for their relatively low-energy but high-nutrient profile

You can even mix every class into a single salad or combine all with meat or fish or poultry or eggs or cheese to make a single stew or casserole.

In the "Phytochemicals and Bioactive Compounds," section of this chapter we'll talk about which are the most concentrated sources of unconventional nutrients, and how these bioactive compounds appear to offer cancer protection.

fruits

Botanically, a fruit is any seed-containing part of the plant. Fruits include apples, apricots, blueberries, cherries, cranberries, figs, grapefruits, grapes, kiwi, lemons, limes, mangoes, melons, nectarines, oranges, papayas, peaches, pears, pineapples, plums, raspberries, and strawberries. Fruits are less easily categorized than vegetables, but they can be divided loosely into some classes:

- **citrus fruits:** oranges, grapefruits, lemons and limes, tangerines, tangelos
- **berries:** raspberries, strawberries, blackberries
- **melons:** watermelon, cantaloupe, squash (pumpkins, zucchini, etc.)

But those categories leave out such fruits as peaches, which come from the same family as plums, apricots, cherries, and nectarines, and have a similar nutritional profile; apples, which come from the same family as pears, tomatoes, pineapples, breadfruit, cassava, dates, figs, avocados, olives, and a whole rainbow of other fruits.

And nearly everything from apricots to papaya to zucchini can be dried and eaten, but there are a few we eat dried so commonly that the dried forms have their own names (raisins and prunes, for example). Others are more often eaten dried (dates and figs), though they can be eaten right off the tree. Drying concentrates the energy in them considerably, but shouldn't drastically affect their nutrient profile. Some dried fruits are treated with chemicals such as sulphur dioxide to preserve color. You may decide you don't want to eat these, but such chemicals should not occur at harmful levels except for those individuals sensitive to these chemicals. Even sun-dried tomatoes can make for a sweet, convenient snack, if you're so inclined.

micronutrient compounds: vitamins, minerals, and unconventional nutrients

For as long as humans have walked the earth, plant chemicals, or phytochemicals, have formed the basis of medicine and pharmacology in every culture. Everything from folk remedies, such as teas, poultices, and energy-enhancing preparations, to powerful drugs, such as morphine, cocaine, digitalis and quinine, are based on plant-derived, biologically active compounds. In many respects, these biologically active compounds have occupied their own separate realm—at least in our culture. For most in our culture, food has always been food—even if Mom's chicken soup did help your cold—and medicine was medicine. Certainly we have always understood that good nutrition often makes for good health ("an apple a day," and so on), but we have always for the most part maintained the distinction between medicinal plants and food plants. Often, this is with good reason—medicinal plants can be potentially toxic and deadly, and need to be used with skill and knowledge.

But our broad, cultural view that food is just food and that one source of protein or fat, for example, can be exchanged for another (as we would rarely do with medicines) is fraught with inaccuracy and myth. Foods can be medicinal, and nutrient foods can be some of the best preventive medicine you can buy.

All vegetables and fruits, depending upon the variety, the soil, and conditions in which they are grown, as well as other factors, will have somewhat different nutritional profiles. A carrot from a farm in California may be nutritionally quite different from one grown in your backyard in Georgia or Iowa or Maine. The famous flavor of the onion from Vidalia, Georgia owes as much to its breed as to the soil and conditions in which it's grown.

(See the AICR Guide to Vitamins, and the AICR Guide to Minerals tables in this chapter for an at-a-glance breakdown on which vegetables and fruits are strongest in which vitamins and minerals, and what these vitamins and minerals do for us in brief.[32])

Almost all vegetables and fruits are quite low in fat, and all are loaded with their own peculiar array of biochemicals. (See also the table on Phytochemicals, page 201.)

Most of the vitamins and minerals we get on a daily basis can be obtained entirely through plant or vegetable sources, whether it's vitamin E from vegetable oils; vitamin A through carotenoids; vitamin C through berries, green, leafy vegetables, citrus, or tomatoes; or vitamin B_{12} from fortified soy products or through the fermentation of vegetable matter in the gut. The same is true of most of the minerals we receive—although in some cases, those from animal sources take fewer metabolic steps to convert into the forms most immediately useful to the body. These more conventionally understood nutrients have considerable "biological activity," and

---

[32] These tables also include animal sources of these vitamins and minerals.

should be talked about before we delve too far into "bioactive compounds," since they are the foundation of cancer-fighting nutrition.

vitamins

As noted above, the notion began to evolve in the 1980s that consuming levels of certain vitamins and minerals in whole food form that are far beyond the minimal levels of the RDAs could help in the fight against many chronic diseases, but particularly against cancer. Those vitamins in particular that have emerged to interest cancer-prevention researchers since that time—and those that have been most closely scrutinized—are:

- the carotenoids (which are plant precursors of vitamin A, or retinol)
- retinol, or preformed vitamin A itself;
- vitamin C
- folate (also known as folic acid)
- vitamin B$_{12}$
- vitamin E

It is important to remember that while each of these different vitamins appears to have proven cancer-fighting potential, it also seems to be *how they work together* (e.g., not in supplement form)—and their synergy with the many other micronutrients that are found in *whole* nutrient foods—that gives them their power to fight against cancer. Examples include the carotenoids and vitamin C.

retinol, or pre-formed vitamin A

Retinol—or preformed vitamin A (usually derived from animal foods)—is a fat-soluble vitamin. Retinol is fundamental to normal cell differentiation, the maintenance of epithelial tissues, night vision, and immune response. Vitamin A deficiency is the leading cause of blindness in developing countries, and affects about half a million children worldwide each year. Low vitamin A intake also decreases resistance to infections such as measles, and increases the morbidity and mortality rates from these diseases in children. It would appear from all available evidence that the best way to boost immune response is to eat lots of vegetables and fruits. If your immune system is working at top form, then all disease is less likely and the virtuous cycle of health, good health, and more good health will result.)

However, excessive intake of retinol from overuse of supplements is toxic and can cause damage to the liver and cell membranes.

Unlike vitamin E or the carotenoids (from which animal bodies, including ours, synthesize retinol), retinol is not an antioxidant.

what role does retinol play in stopping cancer before it starts?

Because of its role in cell differentiation, there has been considerable interest in how retinol may affect cancer risk. Unfortunately, many of the studies of retinol in the past did not separate the preformed vitamin from its precursors, the carotenoids. Still, there is a considerable amount of evidence pertaining to the relationship between retinol and the risk of cancer of a number of sites, and it does not appear to point to retinol by itself as having a very strong relationship. In studies of bladder, lung, stomach, breast, and cervical cancers that separated preformed vitamin A from its plant precursors, there was no clear cut evidence that the retinol (as opposed to the carotenoids) had any appreciable effect in reducing cancer risk.

Since retinol only comes from animal sources, and since our own bodies can synthesize more than adequate amounts from plant sources, the take-home message on vitamin A seems to be, "Eat your vegetables."

the carotenoids

If you've seen the fiery hues of autumn leaves, a carrot, sweet potato, or even algae, you've seen carotenoids, which are pigments synthesized by plants but not animals. They are widespread in nature—there are at least six hundred of them, but they fall into basic categories.

They are fat-soluble compounds known as xanthophylls (carotenoids containing oxygen), carotenes (hydrocarbon carotenoids), or lycopene. (Do you need to remember all these names? No. The important things to remember are the names of the foods that contain them—and to eat plenty of them.)

Some carotenoids are converted to vitamin A, which is required for growth and the normal development and differentiation of tissues. It has also been suggested that carotenoids act as antioxidants in tissues, deactivating free radicals.

Carotene is the most abundant carotenoid. It is found notably in orange vegetables and fruits, such as carrots, sweet potatoes, pumpkin, cantaloupe, apricots, mangoes, and in dark green, leafy vegetables, such as kale, spinach, collard greens, and chicory. Beta-carotene is the most common carotene and the most widespread of all the carotenoids, which explains to some degree why it has been the most studied, but it is not necessarily the most important. Its appearance in the bloodstream (serum levels) can be a relative measure—unless you happen to be taking supplements—of how rich in carotenoids your diet is overall. While some of the studies of beta-carotene (using supplements as the source) and cancer have offered up conflicting results (more cancer cases rather than fewer), most researchers still consider it a valuable cancer-fighting nutrient. The conflicting results of research may partly indicate the overall nutritional poverty of isolated nutrients. Such findings may also indicate that it takes a host of carotenoids working together to provide protection. Another possibility is that a body that gets an adequate dietary complement of carotenoids simply has no need or use for those added in supplementation.

Beta-carotene is the main precursor of vitamin A from plant sources; other carotenoids that have vitamin A activity are cryptoxanthin and alpha-carotene. Carrots are a rich source of alpha-carotene, and avocado and pumpkin also contain appreciable amounts. Cryptoxanthin is found in large amounts in mangoes, persimmon, red peppers, and pumpkin. Consumption of oranges and orange juice can contribute a large proportion of dietary cryptoxanthin.

The predominant carotenoids in spinach, kale, and other greens are the xanthophylls; lutein is the major xanthophyll carotenoid.

Lycopene is found in tomatoes and tomato products, as well as in watermelon, pink grapefruit, and guava.

Carotenoid absorption in the small intestine is relatively inefficient (only 10 to 30 percent of what is eaten is actually absorbed into the bloodstream—but just because it's not absorbed into the bloodstream doesn't mean the body and gut flora don't have other ways of using it). Absorption decreases as carotenoid intake increases or as fat intake decreases, yet another way a no-fat diet would harm you.

High levels of beta-carotene in the diet or blood have been associated with a decreased risk of coronary heart disease in men in at least three studies in this country. Carotenoids are not toxic, even when ingested in very large amounts for weeks, although very high intakes may cause yellowing of the skin.

what role do carotenoids play in stopping cancer before it starts?

While it's impossible, at this date, to say precisely how carotenoids protect against cancers, it is evident from the abundant studies that they do. How they actually do it may be through a number of mechanisms working together. Perhaps most important is their antioxidant capability. Carotenoids are efficient quenchers of reactive oxide molecules and can directly scavenge free radicals. Individual carotenoids have been shown to have variable antioxidant activity—lycopene, for example, exhibits superior antioxidant ability to that of beta-carotene or lutein.

Another theory about the way carotenoids fight cancer has to do with the formation of retinol, or vitamin A. Retinol plays a key role in the regulation of epithelial cell differentiation—epithelial cells being those that line the surfaces of the body's various tissues and therefore spend a lot of time differentiating. Because lack of proper differentiation is a central feature of cancer cells, adequate vitamin A (from any source) may help avoid the development of cancer by helping to promote normal cell differentiation.

There is also evidence that beta-carotene and alpha-carotene may enhance certain aspects of the immune response, and that carotenoids as a group enhance the communication between cells, facilitating normal gene expression. It may prove that all these theories about different cancer-fighting mechanisms are correct. In any case, what's clear is that carotenoids together are a cancer-fighting powerhouse.

vitamin C

Unlike the carotenoids or vitamin E, vitamin C is a water-soluble vitamin. Although many supplements are entirely ascorbic acid, vitamin C appears in foods (and some supplements) in two forms. Ascorbic acid is one, and the "other" vitamin C is dehydroascorbic acid (the oxidized form). Vitamin C is destroyed or lost from food as a result of heat, oxidation, or cooking in large amounts of water, which, as it's water-soluble, causes it to be drained away.

Vitamin C is an essential nutrient and so we must maintain dietary levels of it so that our bodies can keep up a usable pool of it for all our vital functions, which includes facilitating the use of calcium for the building of bones and blood vessels. It also enhances the absorption of the forms of iron we get in plant foods (nonheme iron), which may in turn help to prevent iron-deficiency anemia. Vitamin C is also involved in the healing of wounds, immune response, and other metabolic functions. Vitamin C may also help prevent coronary heart disease by reducing the degree of oxidation of serum cholesterol, which can lead to clogged arteries. Two out of three recent studies in this country have shown a decreased risk of coronary heart disease with higher intakes of vitamin C. An adequate intake of vitamin C is essential to prevent scurvy.

Although many of us associate vitamin C with colds and may take large doses of it when we feel a cold coming on, the use of supplemental megadoses doesn't really demonstrate any clear benefit in either preventing colds or shortening their duration. At daily doses of more than 1,500 mg, more than half may remain unabsorbed in the intestine. A maximum body pool of vitamin C is thought to be reached with intakes of about 100 to 200 mg per day. This is one of those cases where the body needs and uses a certain amount, then gets rid of what's left over. As with carotenoids, smokers generally have lower dietary intakes of vitamin C than nonsmokers as well as lower intakes of their richest sources: vegetables and fruits. But the differences are only partly explained by lower intakes. Somehow, smoking interferes with the body's metabolism of these vital nutrients.

Some controversial research suggests that such megadoses of vitamin C may actually have adverse health effects, including kidney stone formation, gastric distress, altered vitamin B_{12} metabolism, and iron overload, but such potentially toxic effects of vitamin C are disputed. Still, vitamin C, in conjunction with the carotenoids and other vitamins, minerals, and bioactive compounds that come in the nutrient food package, may play a role in stopping colds before they start simply because a healthier you will have a stronger immune response and be less susceptible to infection.

what role does vitamin C play in stopping cancer before it starts?

Vitamin C is an important component of the antioxidant defense system and protects against damage from free radicals. In addition, vitamin C's role in the immune response may enhance the immune system's ability to keep the cells under surveillance for the formation of tumors. It plays a fundamental role in the formation of collagen, which is the essential, fibrous component of "basement" membranes, the foundation for the epithelial cells mentioned above that line the digestive, respiratory, urinary, and reproductive tracts, all potential cancer sites. Collagen is also fundamental to skin and other connective tissue. Because of vitamin C's role in collagen formation, a deficiency of vitamin C might affect the integrity of intracellular walls and may allow tumors to go unchecked; or may inhibit tumor encapsulation.

Perhaps vitamin C's most important function in fighting cancer is that it's the single most abundant water soluble antioxidant in the body. It is unique among antioxidants in that it can be regenerated when oxidized (or the body can render it stable again). Vitamin C can detoxify carcinogens and block damage to DNA through this antioxidant action. It also scavenges and reduces nitrite, which in turn reduces the likelihood of nitrites undergoing nitrosation and forming of potentially carcinogenic N-nitroso compounds.

folate and vitamin B_{12}

Pteroylglutamic acid, more readily known as folate or folic acid, gets its much-easier-to-pronounce name from its abundance in foliage, particularly green leafy vegetables. Vitamin B_{12} is synthesized by gut flora but you also get it from eating animal foods. Traces are sometimes found in plant foods. For those who eat no animal products (meat, dairy, or eggs) fortified cereals or soy products should be used. The latest RDAs call for 2.4 micrograms for all adults and specifically for those over 50. That recommendation includes taking supplements of B_{12} for older people, since some older adults have trouble absorbing B_{12} from food sources.

Research into folic acid and its role in the cancer process is relatively new and ties in perhaps with the comparatively recent findings that tie dietary deficiencies in folic acid to birth defects. Folic acid, along with vitamin B_{12}, is part of the body's production line that creates red blood cells, and so a deficiency in either can lead to folate anemia. It is now quite clear that pregnant women and all women of childbearing age need more folic acid in order to prevent neural tube defects (such as spina bifida) in their babies. Current recommendations are for 400 micrograms for all adult men and older women. It is recommended that women of childbearing age take supplements of 400 micrograms of folic acid daily, and pregnant women should take 600 micrograms daily. Despite the richness of various foods in folates (half a cup of cooked spinach contains about 130 micrograms and an orange contains about 45 micrograms), diets typically consumed in industrialized countries are low in folate, and so a recent law in this country requires that many grain products be fortified with folate.

In addition to helping out with the metabolism of iron and building red blood cells, folic acid plays a leading role in the creation of new cells throughout the body. It does this by assisting in the synthesis and reproduction of purines, the chemicals that make up DNA and RNA, but it also plays a role in the production of lipotropes, the biochemicals that create lipoproteins.

what roles do folate and B$_{12}$ play in stopping cancer before it starts?

Much about how folate and vitamin B$_{12}$ help fight cancer remains to be researched and moved from the realm of theory into realm of fact. Both are crucial to the healthy replication of cells, and deficiencies can lead to fragile chromosomes. Both are also crucial to the synthesis of proteins, particularly lipoproteins, the stuff of which cells are made, as well as cholesterol, both the good and the bad.

It's easy to deduce from this that adequate levels of folate and B$_{12}$ are probably crucial to cancer health, although the research is still so new (and the metabolic processes by which they do their jobs so complex) that facts are yet few.

The lipotropes, or the metabolic compounds that synthesize lipoproteins (of which cell walls are composed) in the liver, may prove to be as important to cancer health as antioxidants, but the process by which they work, and their multitude of interactions with other compounds, make the research into them much more difficult. While we wait for the results of that research, the message is clear: Eat your vegetables early and often.

vitamin E

Vitamin E, like retinol, is a fat-soluble vitamin. Vitamin E is perhaps the most important fat-soluble intracellular antioxidant. Like vitamin C, is not just vitamin E—it comprises at least eight naturally occurring tocopherol and tocotrienol compounds with different biological activities—but only alpha- and gamma-tocopherol appear to be absorbed and retained to any appreciable extent.

Found within the lipid membrane of the body, vitamin E protects polyunsaturated fatty acids in cell membranes from oxidization—oxidization that would otherwise result in the production of malondialdehyde, a suspected mutagen, as well as free radicals that damage cell membranes and DNA—by scavenging oxygen radicals and terminating free radical chain reactions. But once it's done battle with free radicals, vitamin E can be regenerated by other biologically active compounds, including glutathione, an amino acid, and possibly vitamin C.

Vitamin E comes mainly from vegetable oils (including olive, canola, safflower, corn, cottonseed, and soy) and the products made from them, for example, margarine and mayonnaise. Other sources include whole grains, nuts, seeds, and wheat germ (also a good source of folates).

what role does vitamin E play in stopping cancer before it starts?

Vitamin E has potent antioxidant properties, but the evidence of its cancer-fighting abilities is still less than perfectly clear. One mechanism by which vitamin E may reduce cancer risk involves its ability to keep selenium and carotenoids in an active state, thereby enhancing their own antioxidant capacity. Further, vitamin E has been shown to inhibit the formation of nitrosamines, potentially carcinogenic chemicals created from nitrites, which may increase the risk of stomach cancer— however, there appears to be no relationship between vitamin E and stomach cancer. The take-home message on vitamin E would seem to be that it is dependent upon the many different micronutrients of the plant-based portion of our diet, and they, in turn, may depend on it for their cancer-fighting ability.

the take-home message on vitamins

Although it is important that everyone get all the essential vitamins, it is even more important for cancer prevention that we get them through dietary rather than supplementary means—even if that means occasionally getting them from enriched or fortified foods. There is so much interaction between the various micronutrients of these compounds, and so much as-yet-unmapped, potential interaction with the other micronutrients that accompany them in diet, that to avoid vegetables and fruits in favor of supplements appears very foolish.

aicr guide to vitamins

Vitamin (Adult RDA*)	Best sources	Functions
A Retinol, Carotene 800–1000 mcg	Eggs, dark green and yellow vegetables and fruits, low-fat dairy products	Growth and repair of body tissue; immune functions; night vision
B_1 Thiamin 1.0–1.2 mg	Wheat germ, pork, whole and enriched grains, dried beans	Carbohydrate metabolism; appetite maintenance; nerve function; growth and muscle tone
B_2 Riboflavin 1.1–1.3 mg	Low-fat milk products, green leafy vegetables, whole and enriched grains, eggs, meat, poultry, fish	Carbohydrate, fat, and protein metabolism; needed for cell respiration; mucous membranes
B_6 Pyridoxine 1.3–1.7 mg	Fish, poultry, lean meat, whole grains, potatoes	Carbohydrate and protein metabolism; formation of antibodies, red blood cells; nerve function
B_{12} Cobalamin 2.4 mcg	Lean meat, fish, poultry, eggs, low-fat and nonfat milk	Carbohydrate, fat and protein metabolism; maintains nervous system; blood cell formation
Biotin 30 mcg	Egg yolk, cereals, dark green vegetables; also made by microorganisms in intestinal tract	Carbohydrate, fat and protein metabolism; formation of fatty acids; utilization of B vitamins
Folic acid 400 mcg	Broccoli, green leafy vegetables, dried beans, fortified cereals, oranges, nuts	Red blood cell formation; protein metabolism; growth and cell division
Niacin 14–16 mg	Poultry, fish, whole and enriched grains, dried beans and peas	Carbohydrate, fat and protein metabolism; health of digestive system; blood circulation; nerve function; appetite
Pantothenic acid 5 mg	Most plant and animal foods, especially lean meats, whole grains, legumes	Converts nutrients into energy; vitamin utilization; nerve function
C Ascorbic acid 60 mg	Citrus fruits, tomatoes, melons, berries, green and red peppers, broccoli	Wound healing; strengthens blood vessels; collagen maintenance; resistance to infection; healthy gums

(continues)

Vitamin (Adult RDA)	Best sources	Functions
D Cholecalciferol 5–15 mcg 200–600 IU	Egg yolk, fatty fish, fortified milk; also made in skin exposed to sunlight	Calcium and phosphorus metabolism (bone and teeth formation)
E Tocopherol 8-10 mg	Vegetable oil, wheat germ, nuts, dark green vegetables, whole grains	Protects cell membranes and red blood cells from oxidation; may be active in immune function
K 60-80 mcg	Green leafy vegetables, cereal, egg yolk	Formation of blood clotting agents and bone

The Recommended Dietary Allowances (RDAs) shown in this chart are current at the time of writing. However, RDAs are updated regularly, and new recommendations are being incorporated into the new Dietary Reference Intakes (DRIs) which will most likely change the numbers shown here.

Eating plenty of vegetables and fruits is cheap, easy, and good for you, and may significantly lower your risk of cancer and many other chronic diseases. And it would appear that although the recommended minimum of five servings a day is good, this is one of those cases where more is indeed better.

So, how many servings have you had today? Have a few more just to make sure your cancer protection is at its best.

minerals

Although there are many minerals and trace elements that we must have in our diets, there are four that are of particular interest in stopping cancer before it starts. They are calcium (explored with vitamin D here), selenium (both of which may help reduce cancer risk), and iron and iodine. Excess iron or iodine may increase some cancer risk, while deficient levels of intake may also increase cancer risk. Appropriate levels of both these nutrients (and many others) would appear to allow or even enhance the body's ability to maintain its cancer surveillance and protective mechanisms at optimum levels, given good dietary intake of plenty of cancer-fighting nutrient foods.

These are all essential nutrients, and all are available through plant sources, but animal foods may provide more convenient or more readily absorbed forms.

calcium and vitamin D

Most of us associate calcium with strong bones and teeth. While it is essential to the skeletal structure, it has many other important functions, such as in nerve and muscle activity. It plays a variety of roles in the control of cell proliferation and differentiation, which is why it becomes of interest in cancer prevention.

Although low-fat milk and other dairy products are perhaps the best known and easiest sources of calcium, small fish that are eaten with the bones, such as sardines and canned salmon, are also good sources of calcium (as well as iodine). But vegetables can also be a significant source of dietary calcium—raw broccoli, for example, has about 120 mg of calcium in every quarter pound or cup-sized serving. Some vegetables—spinach and some other leafy green vegetables—for example, contain compounds called oxalates, and some grains, notably wheat, contain compounds called phytates, both of which can slightly inhibit the absorption of calcium. This doesn't mean you should eat less of them, it only means you should make sure you get your calcium from as wide a variety of sources as possible.

Vitamin D is essential to the metabolism of calcium as well as phosphorus, and in many respects, because of the role it plays in regulating metabolism, should be considered more as a hormone. Milk in this country is fortified with vitamin D, but our "natural" source of vitamin D is through exposure to sunlight. Older people, particularly seniors, may need more vitamin D than younger people, as they tend to spend less time overall in the sun. Recent studies indicate that most Americans probably do not get enough calcium, so the immediate take-home message on calcium is to eat more bone-containing fish products, more calcium-rich vegetables, and more low-fat milk products, such as yogurt. An hour's walk in the sun will not only help your energy balance and your overall physical fitness, but it will also allow your body to make more vitamin D. (Sunblock won't affect vitamin D synthesis.)

Research shows that vitamin D may work with other nutrients to fight disease. It's been known for years that some vitamins and minerals work better when other nutrients are present. Vitamin E improves the body's use of vitamin A. Vitamin C enhances the absorption of iron. Many of the B vitamins work together, so a deficiency of one usually affects the work of several others. Perhaps the best known nutrient interaction is that of calcium and vitamin D. Vitamin D is critical for the absorption of calcium and the normal deposition of the mineral into bone. Today, scientists are also looking at the way vitamin D and calcium work together as a promising area of diet and cancer research.

"Most studies of the relationship of vitamin D and calcium to the incidence of cancer have focused on one nutrient or the other, but not on both together," says Dr. Richard Davies, Professor of Surgery at the New Jersey Medical School and Director of Surgery at the Hackensack Medical Center. Which is why we've grouped them together here, rather than isolating vitamin D in the vitamin section. Dr. Davies is using an AICR grant to investigate how vitamin D regulates calcium levels in colon cells. Calcium is known to influence cell division in the colon, and several studies have shown that calcium may provide protection against colon cancer.

In his research, laboratory animals are exposed to a colon cancer causing agent and are then divided into two groups—one group receiving vitamin D and one group not. "Cells in the early stages of cancer development are extracted from the colon and studied," Dr. Davies says. "We have already determined that the levels of calcium in these cancer cells has been altered, and we now want to determine if vitamin D affects the level of calcium present," he says. "Once we know more about how calcium and vitamin D interact, we can begin research on colon cancer biomarkers—biological signs which help identify those at high risk for cancer because of the way their bodies handle calcium."

vitamin D and prostate cancer

No firm links have yet been discovered between diet and prostate cancer, but David Feldman, M.D., believes at least one dietary nutrient—vitamin D—may play a role in this second most common cancer in men. Supported in part by a grant from AICR, he is investigating whether vitamin D deficiency increases the risk of developing prostate cancer and promotes its growth.

Dr. Feldman, a professor in the endocrinology division at Stanford University School of Medicine, says that vitamin D affects the growth and development of several types of cells, including prostate cells. "Our work has shown that normal and cancerous prostate cells have vitamin D receptors, indicating they are target cells that can respond to vitamin D," he explains. "We also have found that vitamin D in its active form dramatically inhibits the growth of normal and cancerous prostate cells in a lab dish."

Dr. Feldman is now investigating whether what works in the lab dish will work in mice injected with human prostate cancer cells. Early results indicate a slight benefit when the mice receive vitamin D supplements, although not as dramatic as that observed in the test tube. "I don't think vitamin D will be a cure for prostate cancer, or even a preventative," he says. "What it realistically may do is help slow down the growth of a tumor."

Before vitamin D can be used to treat humans, scientists will have to establish its effectiveness in the body and determine the optimal dose. Excessive levels of vitamin D can be harmful. "We're at the beginning of the story here," Dr. Feldman says. "It's very promising, but there's a long way to go."

promise for treating skin cancer

The effects of vitamin D and calcium on squamous cell carcinoma (SCC), a common type of skin cancer, are the subjects of an AICR grant at the Veterans Administration Medical Center at the University of California in San Francisco. According to the lead researcher, Daniel D. Bikle, M.D., Ph.D., "we've recently discovered that some of the genes which influence cell growth and differentiation, and thus the cancer process, can be turned on and off by exposing normal skin cells to different concentrations of calcium and vitamin D."

"The interaction of vitamin D and calcium is critical to the work I'm doing," Dr. Bikle says. "Vitamin D is the principle regulator of calcium activity in the body, and much of what vitamin D does is mediated by calcium," he adds. "They tend to control each other's levels and work together in the cell changes that are critical to the cancer process."

"It's not inconceivable that one day vitamin D could be used to treat patients at high risk for skin cancer from ultraviolet radiation," says Dr. Bikle. "That's our biggest hope for the future of research on calcium and vitamin D interactions—that these nutrients may eventually be used to prevent and treat cancer."

vitamin D may protect against breast cancer

When we hear about dietary changes to fight breast cancer, most often the focus is on lowering the fat in our diets. Now, new research presented at the AICR research conference on diet and breast cancer suggests that getting enough vitamin D and calcium may also play a role in lowering breast cancer risk.

The effects of these two nutrients on breast cancer development are being investigated by Dr. Harold L. Newmark of the Laboratory of Gastrointestinal Cancer Research at the Memorial Sloan-Kettering Cancer Center and adjunct professor in the Rutgers University Laboratory for Cancer Research. In laboratory animals that had been fed high fat diets and that had developed breast cancer, Dr. Newmark found tumor development was inhibited by increasing the amount of vitamin D and calcium in the animals' diets. Preliminary experiments indicate that these two nutrients may be most effective in reducing breast cancer risk when given to animals during adolescence, a period when their breast cells are growing and changing rapidly.

early eating habits may be important

According to Dr. Newmark, dietary influences on breast cancer in humans may also be most important during the development period of the mammary gland. "Between the ages of eleven and twenty-four, girls and young women seem to be at high risk for damage to DNA that may cause tumors later," he says. Cancers diagnosed later in life may begin during this critical period.

Statistics show that most young women ages 11 to 24 get less than one-third the RDA of vitamin D and only half the RDA of calcium. The new DRI (Dietary Reference Intake) for calcium is 1300 mg for ages 9 to 18, and 1000 mg for adults from age 19 to 50. Dr. Newmark compares breast cancer with osteoporosis, a bone condition that may be intensified by dietary deficiencies of calcium and vitamin D during puberty and adolescence. This is a primary reason it's recommended that girls and women 11 to 24 years old eat more of these nutrients.

how to get more vitamin D

Although scientific studies have not confirmed a link between vitamin D and breast cancer, eating the recommended amount of this nutrient each day is important for good health. One of the best food sources is low fat, vitamin D-fortified milk. Don't count on other dairy products like cheese and yogurt—they aren't typically made with vitamin D-fortified milk. Skim and low-fat varieties of dairy products are also an excellent source of calcium.

what role do calcium and vitamin D play in stopping cancer before it starts?

There is some evidence that diets high in calcium and particularly vitamin D are protective against breast and prostate cancers, but also cancers of the colon and rectum. Exactly what the mechanism is for the protective effect is unclear—it may be that the protective effect has more of a relationship to the complex interactions of these nutrients with other dietary micronutrients.

While calcium supplements may be beneficial to those who are at high risk for osteoporosis, calcium, as with all other dietary micronutrients, is best obtained through dietary means as much as possible. Vitamin C, magnesium, and other nutrients obtained mostly through plant foods, all have a combined effect that cannot be duplicated by supplementation. The effects of other bioactive compounds in this multifaceted process cannot be underestimated. The bottom line? Eat your vegetables and fruits, get D-fortified milk, and get out in the sun (in reasonable amounts and using an effective sunscreen—skin cancer is not our goal).

selenium

Selenium is a trace element found mainly in the germ of grains and in meat and fish. Thought by many to be an antioxidant in its own right, it has no antioxidant properties alone but acts as a co-factor for an enzyme called glutathione peroxidase that protects against oxidative tissue damage. The current RDA for selenium is 55 to 70 mcg a day, but studies show that Americans on average get about twice this much (which may correlate with eating lots of meat). Selenium can have toxic effects if we get too much of it, so this is another case where using supplements is probably a bad idea. A daily dose of about 5 mg can probably cause selenium poisoning.

what role does selenium play in stopping cancer before it starts?

There is some evidence that diets high in selenium may decrease risk of lung cancer. Smokers have lower levels of selenium, but it isn't clear whether this is because they tend to have a lower intake of selenium-containing foods, or if it results from smoking impairing the metabolism of selenium. Experiments have been adjusted for smoking, and still seem to show a protective association. There also seems to be some indication that diets high in selenium may decrease risk for stomach, liver, and thyroid cancers, but it is difficult to draw concrete conclusions.

As with most of the other dietary micronutrients, selenium plays an important, if supporting, role in stopping cancer before it starts. The intake of selenium in the diet should be through low fat foods and whole grains, and it should be joined with high intake of other dietary micronutrients through a diet full of vegetables and fruits.

iron

Iron plays a central role in cell metabolism and growth, and is a fundamental part of red blood cells and their manufacture. Its two main dietary sources are animal and plant foods, and the form most immediately usable to the human body comes from animal-based foods—known as heme iron—and it's most usable because the animals have already metabolized plant-derived iron. It is, however, entirely possible to get plenty of dietary iron without eating animal-based foods at all, and there are ways to improve your body's metabolism of plant-derived iron—nonheme iron. The easiest is to have your iron with vitamin C—for example, have cooked spinach with tomatoes or stewed tomatoes. Some iron can also be had by cooking in unenameled iron cook ware (sauté your spinach and tomatoes together in an iron skillet with some basil).

Where increased cancer risk may arise is that iron is also involved in oxidative metabolism within cells, and is a component of a number of enzymes with diverse roles. Iron can catalyze the generation of free radicals, which cause oxidative damage to specific cell components, including DNA, protein and membrane lipids—remember, iron rusts. But the body strictly regulates iron metabolism to reduce the likelihood of oxidative damage—most iron in living tissues is bound to proteins that prevent its involvement in free radical generation. The body knows it must have iron, but also knows that it has to keep a close watch on it.

Iron-deficiency anemia is common throughout the world, particularly among children and women of childbearing age, and the RDAs for iron may prevent diseases of deficiency but may in some cases be inadequate for all of the functions that utilize iron. This may be particularly true of growing bodies because of iron's role in growth and metabolism. (Does this mean you should take supplements? In some cases, as in adolescent girls, your doctor may recommend them, but in most cases, the best route is to eat fish regularly, along with plenty of the leafy green and other vegetables rich in iron, and to make sure that you get adequate vitamin C.) Women need about 25 percent more iron than men, and our bodies' overall need for iron depends upon whether our dietary iron comes from plant or animal sources. Most likely, it will come from both. If it comes mostly from vegetables, then we need more. If it comes mostly from meat, fish, or poultry, then we need less.

what role does iron play in stopping cancer before it starts?

There is some evidence that diets high in iron may increase the risk of liver and colorectal cancers. Evidence on other cancers is inconclusive. Experimental studies on rats found that iron deficiency (something you want to avoid) inhibited the development of liver tumors, while overload (another something you want to avoid) enhanced carcinogenesis in mice.

The problem most people have, however, isn't too much iron but too little. The World Health Organization has identified iron-deficiency anemia as a worldwide health concern, a problem in industrialized countries as well as developing countries, although the dietary reasons for the problem may differ between developing countries and industrialized ones.

The recommendation for iron would appear to be to try to get as much as you possibly can through dietary means and ensure that growing children have plenty in their diets (most breakfast cereals are fortified with iron, but read labels—some may have only 10 percent of the RDA while others can have as much as 90 to 100 percent). And make sure that you get plenty of all the other dietary micronutrients, particularly vitamin C, that will help your body absorb and utilize the iron. See the AICR Guide to Minerals for sources.

iodine

Seafoods and seaweed are the only reliable dietary sources of iodine, although many plant foods will, depending upon the iodine-content of the soil in which they are grown, contain varying amounts of iodine. Iodine is an essential nutrient, and most salt in this country is iodized. Iodized salt may be your only dietary source of iodine if you are not a fish or seafood eater, so make sure that the salt you buy contains iodine—some, particularly gourmet sea salts, do not.

Iodine forms part of the hormones that are involved in the maintenance of the metabolic rate, cellular metabolism, and the integrity of connective tissue (collagen). In a developing fetus, iodine is essential for the construction of the nervous system—severely deficient mothers are likely to give birth to infants who suffer from mental retardation and other neuromuscular disorders collectively known as iodine deficiency disorders.

what role does iodine play in stopping cancer before it starts?

Most of the evidence on iodine and cancer risk has to do with thyroid cancer. There is evidence that both iodine excess and deficiency may increase the risk of thyroid cancer, but these may be two different types of cancer. Iodine deficiency may increase the risk of certain rare cancers.

In countries where salt iodization programs have been implemented, the incidence of, and mortality rates from, thyroid cancer show contrasting trends: Rates have declined in Switzerland, but not other areas. Iodine deficiency is thought to act indirectly via hormonally mediated pathways, which would likely indicate a role for other dietary micronutrients in the utilization and metabolism of iodine. Diets deficient in iodine probably increase the risk of thyroid cancer.

Excessive long-term intakes of iodine (over one hundred times the RDA) can block the uptake of iodine by the thyroid, leading to goiter. In four case-control studies, high intakes of iodine-rich foods, such as seafood, have been associated with an increased risk of thyroid cancer. Ecological and experimental data also support this association. So while iodine is crucial for survival, we should be careful not to overload iodine in our diets.

the take-home message on minerals

Although it is crystal clear that proper dietary intake of essential minerals is crucial to good health, it is not completely clear whether or exactly how the minerals we've discussed increase or decrease cancer risk. Your best bet for optimum cancer protection is to make sure your diet contains plenty of the vegetables and fruits that contain these minerals. We get iodine from a variety of sources, crops grown near the sea or in iodine-rich soil and dairy products among them. Because of iodine-fortified salt, iodine deficiency is rare. So when you use salt in cooking, make sure it's iodized (but don't oversalt). Use dairy products regularly or use a calcium supplement.

aicr guide to minerals

MINERAL (ADULT RDA)	BEST SOURCES	FUNCTIONS
Calcium 1000–1200 mg	Low-fat or nonfat milk products, calcium fortified orange juice and bread, salmon with bones	Support of bones, teeth, muscle tissue; regulates heartbeat, muscle action, nerve function, blood clotting
Chromium (No RDA)	Cheese, whole grains, meat, peas, beans	Needed for glucose metabolism (energy); increases effectiveness of insulin, muscle function
Copper (No RDA)	Nuts, dried beans, oysters, cocoa powder	Formation of red blood cells, pigment; needed for bone health
Iodine 150 mcg	Seafood, iodized salt	Function of thyroid gland, which controls metabolism
Iron 10–15 mg	Meat, fish, poultry, organ meats, beans, whole and enriched or fortified grains, green leafy vegetables	Formation of hemoglobin in blood and myoglobin in muscle, which supply oxygen to cells
Magnesium 310–420 mg	Nuts, green vegetables, whole grains, dried beans	Enzyme activation; nerve and muscle function; bone growth
Manganese (No RDA)	Nuts, whole grains, vegetables, fruits	Bone growth and development; sex hormone production; cell function
Phosphorus 800–1200 mg	Meat, poultry, fish, eggs, low-fat milk products, beans, whole grains	Bone development; carbohydrate, fat and protein utilization
Potassium (No RDA)	Vegetables, fruits, beans, bran cereal, low-fat milk products	Fluid balance; controls activity of heart muscle, nervous system
Selenium 55–70 mcg	Seafood, lean meat, grains, eggs, chicken, garlic	Fights cell damage from oxidation
Zinc 12–15 mg	Lean meat, eggs, seafood, whole grains, lowfat milk products	Taste and smell sensitivity; regulation of metabolism; aids in healing

phytochemicals and bioactive compounds

If you saw them listed as ingredients on a cereal box you might be alarmed: isoflavones, terpenes, indoles, phenolic acids, and bioflavonoids. But these strange names, which sound a lot like things you might wash your floor with, aren't artificial additives, they're naturally occurring chemicals found in foods like fruits, vegetables, and grains, chemicals our bodies use as part of their disease-fighting arsenal. All of these are bioactive, and all of these are phytochemicals. Some have been used for medicinal purposes for centuries. The anti-cancer effects of many of them, however, are only beginning to be explored.

Isothiocyanates, for example, which are found in cruciferous vegetables such as broccoli and cabbage, protect against cancer through their effect on enzymes. Saponins, found in beans and legumes, may prevent cancer cells from multiplying by influencing the genetic material in the cells.

A single tomato or orange contains hundreds, and possibly thousands, of phytochemicals. Indeed, much of the work thus far has been simply cataloging and classifying them.

what role do phytochemicals in stopping cancer before it starts?

Many.

Phytochemicals differ from vitamins and minerals in that they have no conventional nutritional value. Some are antioxidants, protecting against harmful cell damage by oxidation. Others perform different functions that help prevent cancer. Today's laboratory pioneers are still deciphering the many ways phytochemicals in foods may offer front-line defenses against cancer.

One reason scientists are so excited about phytochemicals is their apparent ability to stop a cell's conversion from healthy to cancerous at so many different stages. Indoles, a family of phytochemicals found in cruciferous vegetables, stimulate enzymes that perform many functions. One impact is to make the hormone estrogen less effective, possibly reducing breast cancer risk. Following are some of the specific compounds from the various classes of vegetables and fruits and how they seem to act in cancer prevention.

allium compounds

Allium compounds are found in the allium vegetables, which include onions, garlic, scallions, and chives. It is these compounds that account for the distinctive flavor and aroma of allium vegetables, as well as for the many reported medicinal effects.

Allium compounds may have anticarcinogenic mechanisms involving the enzymatic detoxification systems. Allium vegetables have also been hypothesized to protect against cancer by inhibiting the bacterial conversion of nitrate to nitrite in the stomach. They have antibiotic properties and may act against *Heliobacter pylori,* a cause of ulcers and a known factor for increased risk of stomach cancer.

Allyl sulfides in garlic may decrease the tendency for blood clots to form and reduce total and LDL cholesterol levels, thereby protecting against heart disease. Flavonoids may protect against heart disease by protecting LDL cholesterol from oxidation and by inhibiting platelet aggregation.

dithiolthiones

Dithiolthiones are found in cruciferous vegetables (broccoli, cauliflower, cabbage), as are the isothiocyanates—benzyl isothiocyanate, phenethyl isothiocyanate and sulforaphane. Isothiocyanates are also found in other vegetables and in spices and are produced synthetically.

Dithiolthiones are, like garlic and other allium vegetable-type compounds, sulfur-containing compounds and are thought to protect against cancer by inhibiting enzymes that activate carcinogens or by inducing detoxifying enzymes.

terpenoids

Terpenoids such as D-limonene, found in citrus fruits and cherries, are believed to protect against cancer by inducing the family of enzymes called glutathione transferases. Glutathione is one of the most important intracellular antioxidants,[33] possibly evolving as a molecule that protects cells against oxygen toxicity.

---

[33] Which is not to diminish the importance of the other most important antioxidants, vitamin C, the most important water-soluble antioxidant, or vitamin E, the most important fat-soluble antioxidant. There are many different places and ways in which our bodies use these important compounds.

phytoestrogens

Phytoestrogens, found most richly in soy products (soy milk, tofu), have numerous biological effects. They are antiviral, antiproliferative, and growth inhibiting. Phytoestrogens are weakly estrogenic and can compete with steroid hormones for various enzymes and receptors. They also stimulate production of sex hormone-binding globulin in the liver. In these ways, they may alter hormone metabolism and, by inhibiting growth and proliferation of hormone-dependent cancer cells, may alter cancer risk.

flavonoids

Flavonoids are found in fruits, vegetables, coffee, tea, cola, and alcoholic beverages. Quercetin, campferol, and myricetin are flavonols widely distributed in vegetables and fruits. The richest sources of quercetin are berries, tomatoes, potatoes, broad beans, broccoli, Italian squash (zucchini), and onions, the strongest concentration actually being in onion skin (so throw the skins into the mix when you're making soup or stew and take them out before serving). Radishes, horseradish, kale and endive are relatively high in campferol. Other flavonoids (tangeretin, nobiletin and rutin) are found in citrus fruits.

Other phenolic compounds are found in freshly harvested vegetables and fruits, and in relatively large amounts in teas and wines. Ellagic acid is found in high concentrations in fruits and nuts, specifically in strawberries, raspberries, blackberries, walnuts, and pecans (which sounds like a recipe for dessert tonight). Ellagic acid reduces the genetic damage caused by carcinogens like tobacco smoke or air pollution. It does this by affecting the carcinogen, and also, possibly, by directly protecting the cell's genetic material.

Tofu, soy milk, and other foods made from soybeans are rich in the isoflavones, which may inhibit cancer cell growth and division under some conditions. Since cancer is the result of the cell growth process gone awry, isoflavones may provide a means for switching off the unusual growth.

coffee, tea, and other drinks

It's reasonably easy to apply everything you know about foods to drinks. Soft drinks, with their very high level of refined sugars, are probably best avoided or drunk only in moderation. Diet soft drinks, while they have no sugar, do not really offer anything beneficial and should probably be traded in for other drinks with known value. Some fruit juices, although they can be relatively high in calories, are wonderful sources of vitamin C, but also of other cancer-fighting phytochemicals. Tea, particularly green tea, can have valuable antioxidants.

Some drinks have been linked in the popular press with cancer, so let's take a look at them.

Milk (and dairy products in general) has been linked to a possible higher rate of cancers of the prostate and kidney, although the evidence is mostly inconclusive. Milk is a source of calcium and the best dietary source of vitamin D (which is added to milk). It is also a source of saturated fats, so when drinking milk, go for skim or 1 percent milk.

Coffee is made from the dried and roasted seed of the berry of the coffee tree. It has demonstrated no conclusive link to any cancer, and there is some evidence that it may decrease risk of colorectal cancers, but that evidence is sketchy. There is some sketchy evidence that it may be linked (with other hot drinks) to cancers of the mouth, pharynx, and esophagus, but this has more to do with its being drunk extremely hot than with coffee itself. It should be said, however, that coffee does act as a vasoconstricting stimulant and may increase levels of stress hormones (that may adversely affect immune response), so if you tend towards high blood pressure or have a stressful enough life, there may be no reason artificially to increase your stress.

Coffee has been shown conclusively to have no relationship to breast cancer. It has been shown to be likely to have no relationship to cancers of the stomach, pancreas, and kidney. Any possible increase in cancer risk from coffee comes from drinking very large amounts (5 or more cups per day) on a regular basis. Still, the evidence is sketchy.

Tea is made up of the leaves of tea plants. Green tea, which shows some evidence of reducing the risk of stomach cancer, is produced from tea leaves that have been exposed to high temperatures only long enough to deactivate fermenting enzymes. Black tea is the withered, rolled, fermented, and finally roasted tea leaf. Oolong tea is a semi-fermented tea.

There is some sketchy evidence that tea may increase risk of cancer of the esophagus, but this, as with coffee and other hot drinks, is more a result of its being drunk extremely hot rather than any intrinsic property of the tea itself. Iced tea can be a refreshing alternative to soft drinks. Not only is it considerably less expensive, you can flavor it to your liking with herbs and spices (rosemary, lavender, cloves, cinnamon, lemon or orange zest) that have their own cancer-fighting potential. There are many non-tea herbal teas you can purchase that may offer valuable cancer-fighting phytochemicals in addition to good flavor. You can also make your own with herbs and spices. Check the shelves of your local grocer or your local health food store and see what they have to offer.

Neither tea nor coffee contains much in the way of conventional nutrients, although both contain caffeine.

Soft drinks are usually made from sugar and water and artificial flavorings. Some, particularly colas, have added caffeine. Aside from their ubiquitousness, there is really no reason to drink soft drinks or diet soft drinks when there are so many other things around to drink. If you like your drink to sparkle, you can create your own, much more healthful, soft drinks by mixing one part fruit juice to one part seltzer. By whatever odd quirk of the taste bud, a fruit juice that's been diluted with seltzer doesn't taste watered down. Or you can just drink seltzer water, which may contain some sodium. Read labels.

See *Alcohol*, if you haven't already, in chapter 8.

the take-home message on coffee, tea, and other drinks

As always, limit refined sugars and unneeded fats. There's no reason not to have a soft drink as an occasional treat, or a dollop of honey in your tea on a chilly winter morning, but remember to keep things in balance. Human beings are made up mostly of water, so it's only natural to make water your thirst-quencher of choice.

phytochemicals in cancer treatment

In addition to cancer-prevention, phytochemicals are also being studied in cancer treatment, where they are used in amounts so concentrated they qualify as drugs. Pamela Crowell, Ph.D., an assistant biology professor at Indiana University-Purdue University at Indianapolis, has found that perillyl alcohol, found in cherries and lavender, causes pancreatic tumors to regress in laboratory animals. She says these compounds appear to cause tumor cells to shift to a less malignant type. Perillyl alcohol belongs to a class of phytochemicals called terpenes. Limonene, contained in the peel (zest) of citrus fruits,[34] is one of the best known phytochemicals in this class. In laboratory animals it blocks the development of breast tumors and causes existing tumors to regress.

Taxol, another member of the terpene family, is not found in food, but is a phytochemical already being used in clinical trials. The Food and Drug Administration approved the compound, derived from the relatively rare Pacific yew tree, for treating ovarian cancer in 1992 and breast cancer in 1994. Taxol is now made in a semisynthetic process, so there is no shortage of the drug.

Molecular pharmacologist Susan Band Horwitz, Ph.D., has been studying taxol since the 1970s. It was her laboratory at the Albert Einstein College of Medicine in the Bronx that first determined how taxol works to prevent cell division. Although it is used in very low concentrations, it does have side effects such as hair loss, says Horwitz. She stresses that people and animals have died from ingesting taxol in its natural state. Phytochemicals, like many other chemicals, can be toxic and must be properly formulated and tested before using them in the concentrated forms necessary for cancer treatment.

phytochemical designer foods?

Is an anticancer cocktail brimming with extrastrength phytochemicals soon to be on supermarket shelves? Many experts predict it won't be long before some of the better-known phytochemicals start appearing in pills or packaged foods the way vitamins, calcium, beta-carotene, and other nutrients are now. Indeed, the National Cancer Institute's major foray into phytochemicals was dubbed the Designer Foods Research Project when it was first announced in 1989 by Ritva Butrum, Ph.D., then chief of the NCI's Diet

---

[34] Zest—what a wonderful word. Most of the peel of citrus fruits is bitter and completely unpalatable, although you could probably eat it. The zest, however, which is the porous, colorful, outer part, is delicious and full of limonene. You can use a vegetable peeler to pare off the zest of citrus fruits for use in cooking. Instead of just using the juice of lemons in your iced tea, add the zest to water along with tea. You can also add it to sauces—it has a more delicate flavor than the juice (less acid and less sugar) and really adds the essence of the fruit to your cooking. Be careful to wash your fruits thoroughly, however, as many are waxed before market to give them a longer shelf-life, and although the wax isn't poisonous, there's no reason to add it to your meal.

and Cancer Branch, and now Vice President for Research at the American Institute for Cancer Research. Carolyn Clifford, Ph.D., who directs the program today, says the technology is far ahead of the science at this point.

"You can modify the chemical constituents in food through plant breeding, bioengineering, and food processing, but before we get to that stage we need to know: What compounds? What levels are effective?" says Clifford.

In other words, would megadoses of certain phytochemicals really head off cancer? Could they have harmful side effects?

Does the preventive punch of phytochemicals depend upon dozens or hundreds of them working together in a complex ballet, as they do in foods?

Seattle-based nutritionist Mark Messina, Ph.D., formerly with the NCI, does not endorse the trend toward souped-up cereals or what might be called "phytamin" pills. "I think we should focus our time on getting people to consume the type of diet we already know will reduce cancer risk. The notion of designer foods is in essence trying to supplement your way to good health. It doesn't make up for a bad diet."

the take-home message on phytochemicals

Although cruciferous vegetables and citrus fruits are developing reputations as phytochemical powerhouses, keep in mind that these are simply the most studied foods, and scientists are learning more every day. Eating a variety of vegetables and fruits is more important than concentrating on particular kinds. A variety of these foods will help you get the full gamut of phytochemicals found in nature.

Here are some easy ways of increasing your intake of phytochemicals.

◆ Eat more whole grains. Don't limit your carbohydrate selection to bread, rice, and pasta. Try quinoa, bulgur, barley, kasha, or the more exotic rices, such as wehani and wild rice (which is not, botanically speaking, a true rice) for variety. Once available only in health food stores, most of these grains have become supermarket staples.

◆ Eat a variety of vegetables. Broccoli is very nutritious, but you don't have to eat it every day. Don't forget carrots, cauliflower, leafy greens, winter and summer squashes, green and red peppers, snow peas, red cabbage...the list is endless. Bags of mixed vegetables in

phytochemicals and where to get them

PHYTOCHEMICAL FAMILY	FOOD SOURCES
Allyl Sulfides	Onions, garlic, leeks, chives
Indoles	Cruciferous vegetables (broccoli, cabbage, kale, cauliflower)
Isoflavones	Soybeans (tofu, soy milk)
Isothiocyanates	Cruciferous vegetables
Phenolic Acids (ellagic acid, ferulic acid)	Tomatoes, citrus fruits, carrots, whole grains, nuts
Polyphenols	Green tea, grapes, red grape juice, wine, chocolate
Saponins	Beans and legumes
Terpenes (perillyl alcohol, limonene)	Cherries, citrus fruit peel

the frozen foods section make getting an assortment at a single meal easy. Don't feel you have to eat a wide variety every day; your weekly consumption is what's important.

◆ Eat more fruits. Research shows the average American eats about one serving a day. A glass of juice at breakfast is nice, but how about some bananas, blueberries, or peaches atop your cold or hot cereal? A crisp apple or fragrant orange (or tangerine or clementine or even a grapefruit) as a midday snack or perfectly ripe (or even frozen) strawberries for dessert?

◆ Don't forget herbs and spices. Even though you don't eat much of them, they contain phytochemicals, too. Garlic, hot peppers, basil, parsley, and other fresh and dried herbs add zip to low-fat foods.

◆ Decrease portion sizes of meat, fish, and poultry. You'll naturally eat more grains, vegetables, and fruits if you do. Remove half the filling from an overstuffed deli sandwich. Update a favorite dish by changing the meat-to-vegetable ratio: chicken and pasta casserole with peas can become pea and pasta casserole with chicken. Make Sloppy Joe with ground turkey and textured vegetable protein instead of hamburger.

◆ Explore new foods and new recipes. Tofu is a phytochemical-filled option, but how to prepare it may be a challenge. The same may be true for other unfamiliar offerings in the produce department, like jicama, fennel, tomatillos, daikon, papaya, or passion fruit. Some supermarkets offer recipe cards or fliers to encourage customers to try the more exotic fare. Simply turn to page 227 to check out one of the many new low-fat healthy recipes we've included for how-to's. But don't limit yourself. Experiment.

"Five years ago we didn't know about half the phytochemicals we know of today; five years from now we'll know about that many more," says Dr. Messina. "I think the bottom line with phytochemicals is that they just give us more reasons to consume a plant-based diet."

salt

The famed food writer and gastronome M.F.K. Fisher wrote that any dish that can be improved by the mere addition of salt is probably pretty lousy food. We have as a species a taste for salt, much as we have a taste for sugar. Foods in nature are generally poor sources of sodium and are generally much higher in potassium. It has been suggested that animals and humans have an inbuilt desire for salt as a compensatory mechanism: hence salt licks used by herbivorous animals and the high value placed on salt throughout human history. The word *salary* derives from the Latin word for salt, because salt was sometimes part of the pay of Roman soldiers.

Today, even though salt is still absolutely necessary for survival, salt is everywhere, particularly in the prepared foods we eat. Unless we're sweating in the hot sun all day long and losing whopping amounts of salt, most of us have to be careful about our salt intake because it has been shown again and again to be deadly in large amounts. A recent study showed that high intakes of salt can cause hypertension even in children, and abundant evidence from regions where salt-preserved foods are still eaten in large quantities shows that it can, if eaten chronically in significant amounts, increase the risk of certain cancers considerably.

Since salt is used extensively by the food industry, the diets consumed in developed countries typically include salt in concentrations and volumes far in excess of anything we need. Diets high in salted foods and in salt itself probably increase the risk of stomach cancer.

Salt in diets comes from salt added for preservation, in manufacturing, in cooking, or at the table. Diets become salty only because we make them so—when salt is added as part of processing, designed to preserve food or to make it more attractive. Salt or other forms of sodium is added to a vast range of processed foods. Sodium in processed meat such as bacon, ham and sausage is usually 200 to 600 mg per 3-ounce serving. The volume of sodium in bread may vary between 150 and 400 mg per slice. Breakfast cereals contain variable amounts of salt: as much as a whopping 400 mg per cup. Snacks such as potato chips, pretzels, and peanuts can be quite salty, and can contain up to 500 mg of sodium per ounce. Read Nutrition Facts labels. Many cheeses, such as cheddar and parmesan, have considerable amounts of added sodium. Processed "lunch boxes" purchased by harried and unwitting parents for consumption by their children can contain as much as 1500 mg of sodium in a single portion.

Sodium deficiency is vary rare even among populations whose intake is very low. So how much sodium do we need? A safe daily intake has been estimated at 500 mg for adults. It has also been argued that average sodium intake is around 10 times the recommendation. The upper *limit* should be around 2400 mg a day, depending upon a person's size, health, and physical activity. Those people subject to heavy and persistent sweating may become depleted, as may individuals suffering chronic diarrhea or renal disease, but they are the exception rather than the rule.

Sodium is identified as an important cause of hypertension and stroke in the amounts present in those diets that include substantial amounts of salted or salty food.

getting salt out of your (and your family's) diet

There are a number of ways you can reduce salt in the foods you prepare, as well as in processed foods:

- First of all, read labels. Don't buy foods that contain large amounts of salt or sodium.
- When buying canned tomatoes or tomato sauce, for example, look for the varieties that contain no salt at all. If you're making pasta sauce, then you can add herbs such as oregano and rosemary instead of salt. This will add flavor as well as important cancer-protective phytochemicals. Then, if you need to, you can salt to taste.
- When cooking processed or preserved foods such bacon or sausage,

you can get rid of at least some of the salt by cooking them in water first. Before frying, fill your skillet about halfway with water, cook the meat in boiling water for several minutes, then pour off the water and brown. You can also use a similar technique in the microwave.

- When preparing meats, you can leave out the salt and instead use marinades that include anything from lemon juice, wine, and flavored vinegars to lots of herbs and spices, as well as lots of garlic and onions.
- Avoid processed meats, which contain high levels of salt and sugar.
- Avoid processed starchy foods such as some frozen meals, which may contain high levels of salt.
- Avoid conventional snack foods, such as chips and pretzels.
- Use herbs, spices, and other "flavor enhancers" instead of salt.

flavor enhancers that may enhance health

Dr. James Duke, the author of *The Green Pharmacy,* is a man with a mission. A retired botanist for the U.S. Department of Agriculture (USDA), he is interested in cataloging every chemical compound in every plant reported to fight disease—every leaf, seed, peel, pod and root we pop into our mouths.

This task would take several lifetimes to complete, of course, but Duke has made an impressive and promising start. Before his retirement in late 1995, he established the landmark Phytochemical Database for the USDA—a database that lists all the known chemical compounds in more than one thousand edible plants, including the most common herbs and spices consumed. "And I'm still adding to it," says Duke. Each month he culls nearly two dozen scientific journals for information and makes updates in his personal computer. The data will eventually be transferred to the main USDA database, helping scientists figure out the most promising compounds to study for disease protection.

What Duke has gleaned in his decades of research is that many of the herbs and spices we use every day—oregano, orange peel, caraway, turmeric, celery seed, and dozens of others—are sources of cancer-fighting chemicals. Take caraway, for example, the seed that gives rye bread its distinctive flavor. Duke says it contains phytochemicals like carvone, perillyl alcohol, and limonene. Studies suggest the last two may be able to shrink certain tumors; scientists think carvone may as well, because it belongs to the same class of phytochemicals. Limonene, the best studied of this phytochemical trio, is also found in citrus peel, celery seed, cardamom, fennel, spearmint, nutmeg, star anise, and thyme.

Then there's oregano, that essential ingredient in pizza and pasta sauce. A 1992 French study of more than seventy herbs found oregano to be the best source of rosmarinic acid and other closely related antioxidants. "I don't know of a single herb or spice that doesn't have a folk remedy attributed to it—and more often than not they turn out to be fairly accurate once we find out the chemistry that explains the folklore," says Duke, who, in addition to *The Green Pharmacy,* has published fifteen books on the subject. He cites rosemary as an illustration. It's often called the "remembrance" herb. Now studies show that it contains compounds that may be useful in fighting Alzheimer's disease.

The AICR has funded considerable research on promising phytochemicals in natural flavorings, including limonene, curcumin (found in turmeric, a curry spice), coumarin (found in fenugreek, a component of some herbal teas), and organosulfides (found in the allium family of vegetables, which includes garlic and onion). Duke says there's mounting evidence to suggest that these plant compounds work best in combination, not isolation. He believes this synergistic effect is an argument against popping supplements. "I don't believe in a silver bullet in either medicine or in nutrients," he says. "Vitamins and phytochemicals are better taken in their evolutionary context—as they occur in plants—not isolated and out of context."

herbs and spices

What's the difference between an herb and a spice? Herbs are usually the fresh or dried leaves of the plant, while spices are often the ground seeds (but sometimes the bark or stems) of the plant. If you can, always try to use fresh herbs—they can be lots of fun to grow in the garden or on the window sill, and don't take much effort. If you have a reliable means for grinding, buy your spices whole: they'll last longer that way. Some, however, are quite hard, and may be difficult to grind very well. The rule of thumb for herbs and spices of the dried variety is to replace them every New Year's Day, since even though dried, they still lose their flavor and potency over time.

Herbs and spices offer a low-sodium (and cancer-healthy) way to season and transform ordinary foods. Nearly every one of the herbs and spices listed below has at least one valuable chemical that has been associated with cancer prevention and cancer health. Rosemary, for example, has some twenty anti-oxidants, and has shown promise in reducing some tumors.

But what can you do when a recipe calls for herbs and spices you don't ordinarily keep on your shelves?

If you have the money, the kitchen space, and the desire for a taste treat, go ahead and buy a small amount. In fact, always buy spices in small quantities unless you plan to use them up rapidly. Purchasing herbs and spices in bulk, rather than pre-packaged, means you can buy as much or as little as you want. The chart that follows offers advice on what sorts of herbs and spices are commonly used with foods. However, the emphasis in your purchasing and use should be on what you like. If you happen to like rosemary or cumin or nutmeg, use it wherever you want. Don't let these suggestions limit you. Use them as a starting point for discovery.

Keep in mind a few basic principles when using herbs and spices:

- Use what you like (and what your family likes).
- If you're just starting out, experiment until you feel more comfortable choosing compatible flavorings, and select only one or two herbs per dish. This way you can evaluate the flavors—if you throw in everything but the spice rack, you'll likely not be able to tell which combination works and which doesn't.
- You can add garlic or onion (fresh or powdered, cooked or raw) to nearly anything and make it taste better (maybe not your breakfast cereal) but garlic and onion both have fine cancer-fighting properties in addition to tasting good.
- Don't overdo it. Most spices and herbs are quite flavorful (unless they've been sitting on the shelf for years). Start with small amounts. Sniff and taste everything you use. As a rule of thumb, allow about ¼ teaspoon herbs per serving as a starter until you get a feel for the amount that suits your taste.

using herbs and spices

Herbs and Spices	Meat	Poultry	Fish	Soup	Vegetables	Salad
basil	•	•	•	•	•	•
bay leaf	•	•	•	•		
celery seed			•		•	•
chili powder	•	•	•			
chives		•		•	•	•
cloves	•			•		
coriander (seed)	•		•	•		
cumin	•	•				
curry	•	•	•		•	
dill		•	•	•	•	•
fennel (seed)	•		•	•		
ginger	•	•	•	•	•	
mace				•		
marjoram	•	•		•	•	•
nutmeg					•	
oregano	•	•	•	•	•	•
paprika		•	•	•		•
rosemary	•	•	•		•	
saffron		•		•		
sage		•		•		
savory	•			•	•	
tarragon		•		•	•	•
thyme	•	•		•	•	•

hints for using herbs

◆ **Basil:** Goes well with fish, shellfish, and vegetables such as tomatoes, zucchini and eggplant.

◆ **Chives:** Use in fish dishes, soups, salad dressings, and on baked potatoes or steamed vegetables. (Chives taste better when preserved by freezing rather than drying.)

◆ **Dill:** This mild herb is excellent in yogurt sauces, rice dishes and soups. Goes well with fish and vegetables like cucumbers and carrots.

◆ **Oregano:** Essential to Italian cuisine, oregano is found in most tomato sauces and dishes. Use in salad dressings, soups or bean and vegetable dishes. Oregano tastes best dried.

◆ **Parsley:** It's not just sprigs any more. Or it shouldn't be. Use parsley generously to spice up salads, soups, bean dishes, fish and vegetables like tomatoes, artichokes and zucchini. Fresh parsley is usually preferred to dried. Flat-leafed, or Italian parsley, has a slightly different flavor from curly leafed or common parsley. Cilantro, sometimes known as Chinese parsley—which is not parsley at all but fresh coriander—has a flat leaf but a much different flavor from Italian parsley. Use it in everything from salsas to Asian dishes. There is some evidence that parsley, which contains boron and fluorine, can help fight osteoporosis.

◆ **Rosemary:** Use this strong, fragrant herb when making roasted potatoes or chicken, homemade bread, soups, rice and marinades.

◆ **Thyme:** This aromatic herb goes well with poultry, seafood, and many bean and vegetable dishes, including eggplant, tomatoes, mushrooms, squash, and onions.

rosemary

Nutrition-wise cooks know that judicious use of herbs and spices helps provide the flavor needed to cut the fat in recipes. Now scientists are beginning to find an additional role for these flavorings in a healthy diet since phytochemicals found in several popular herbs and spices have been identified as potential sources of cancer protection.

At the University of Illinois Department of Food Science and Human Nutrition, Dr. Keith Singletary has used a grant from AICR to investigate the cancer-protective potential of the herb rosemary. "It's been known for years that rosemary extract has strong antioxidant properties, so we wanted to see how it might affect tumors in animal models and to identify the phytochemicals involved," Dr. Singletary says.

In his experiments, Dr. Singletary used both rosemary extract and a component of rosemary called carnisol. Various levels of these substances were included in the diets of laboratory rats; other laboratory rats received the substances through injection. The animals were exposed to a carcinogen known to cause mammary (breast) cancer and studied to see how the rosemary extract and carnisol might afford protection against mammary DNA damage. "We measured the activity of two liver enzymes which detoxify chemical carcinogens," Dr. Singletary says. "Rosemary extract in the diet and rosemary extract and carnisol administered through injection resulted in a significant enhancement of enzyme activity and less damage to mammary DNA from the carcinogen."

With this information, Dr. Singletary went on to conduct a larger animal study which confirmed the finding that rosemary extract and carnisol hold considerable promise as blocking agents against breast cancer. He notes that other researchers have found that these substances also protect against skin cancer and enhance defense against carcinogenic damage in human lung cells.

What researchers don't know about rosemary is how much must be consumed to achieve cancer protection. "While we don't know the dose-response relationship for rosemary, it is encouraging to know that it provides not only an alternative to fat and salt for flavoring, but also useful phytochemicals that may reduce cancer risk," Dr. Singletary says.

In addition to his rosemary studies, Dr. Singletary is investigating curcumin (a component of the spice turmeric) and phytochemicals in vaccinium fruit (cranberries, blueberries and lingonberries), which appear to enhance cancer-protective enzymes and slow the growth of tumor cells.

the take-home message on rosemary and other herbs

These plant-derived flavorings can offer to your cooking a great deal more than flavoring. They offer the potential for a whole new dimension of cancer-protective additions to your diet. Instead of using salt or fat to enhance the flavor of your food, you can use herbs, and the numbers of ways you can use them are only limited by your imagination. There's the simple and obvious basil and vinegar with your sliced, fresh tomatoes, but for a change of pace, what about ground cumin and coriander on them? Or how about a little cinnamon or rosemary or garlic powder on air-popped popcorn instead of butter and salt? There's virtually a whole rainbow of different herbs and spices you can use. You can use the table in Using Herbs and Spices as a guide, but the important thing is to use what you like. Many herbs, like rosemary and lavender, can be used in teas as well as in flavorings. Next time you're making iced tea, forget the sugar and add into the tea some fresh (or dried) rosemary. And don't just squeeze the juice out of the lemon (a great source of vitamin C), use a vegetable peeler and put some of the lemon rind, the zest—just the outer, yellow part, not the white, pithy part—into the tea as well. It's a great source of D-limonene.

SOY

Soybeans and nearly all of the many products that are made from them have some of the most profoundly unappetizing names in the food universe. Bean curd (or its other name, tofu), textured vegetable protein, tempeh—none of these is very likely to send anyone sailing to the refrigerator on clouds of gustatory anticipation. Even the word soy itself sounds remarkably like *soil.* And soy's most well-known product, soy sauce, which probably has more salt in it than soy itself, tends to conjure up images of *other* foods, or little plastic packets.

It's a shame that this is the case, because aside from being wonderfully versatile (how many other plant products can you name that can range from milk to nuts?), soy is a wonderful source of protein and is also loaded with valuable, potentially important, cancer-fighting phytochemicals.

Phytoestrogens are a case in point. These are hormone-like substances found primarily in foods made from soybeans. Researchers believe they show great promise in blocking critical steps of the cancer process. With the help of grants from AICR, Dr. Stephen Barnes at the University of Alabama at Birmingham has spent the past eight years conducting research on a phytoestrogen called *genistein.* Based on the findings of this research, Dr. Barnes recently obtained a substantial grant from the National Cancer Institute (NCI) to further his work with genistein.

Dr. Barnes's research suggests that genistein acts as an estrogen "antagonist," helping to block cancers related to hormone activity, such as breast or prostate cancer. "Phytoestrogens are very weak estrogens, about a hundred to a thousand times less effective than natural estrogens," explains Dr. Barnes. He describes their possible role in cancer prevention with a baseball analogy: "Even though I'm not much of a baseball player, I'd look quite good playing with six- and seven-year-olds. If I tried to play with professionals, however, I wouldn't look good at all. I'd get in the way of the other players and ruin their plays.

"In the same way, weak phytoestrogens look good in the right circum-stances—they appear to do what natural estrogens do. But in the presence of these natural estrogens, phytoestrogens tend to compete by getting in their way and blocking the estrogen activity related to cancer promotion."

Research conducted under AICR grants allowed Dr. Barnes to delve into the process by which genistein may help fight cancer. He was able to elimi-nate several popular theories about how the phytoestrogen works and can now focus new resources on more promising ideas. One important aim of future studies is to develop compounds similar to genistein for use in can-cer therapy.

While improved cancer treatment is one important outcome of his research, Dr. Barnes is also very interested in the prevention of cancer. One of Dr. Barnes's graduate students recently completed research showing that genistein is ten times more effective at inhibiting cancer growth in nor-mal, noncancerous cells than in cells where cancer growth has already started. "Cancer cells don't seem to be as sensitive to genistein as normal cells are," Dr. Barnes notes.

To obtain more concrete information about genistein's impact on human cancers, Dr. Barnes is currently involved in three clinical trials—two on breast cancer and one on prostate cancer. In the first, thirty-seven healthy pre- and post-menopausal women in San Francisco are consuming diets with and without soy. Researchers are examining their breast fluid for properties that may mean greater risk of breast cancer. In the second trial, at the University of Alabama at Birmingham, forty elderly men with elevat-ed prostate-specific antigen (PSA) levels, which means they may be at risk for prostate cancer, are drinking soy beverages to see if the isoflavones lower the PSA levels.

Should you add soy products to your shopping list? Although the evi-dence so far is only by association, many people in other parts of the world eat soy foods and their risk of illnesses such as cancer and heart disease is much lower than in this country. As with all foods, however, moderation is recommended. Soy foods can be significant sources of fat as well as phytoe-strogens. One ounce of tofu (usually sold in eight ounce packages) has 41 calories and over 2 grams of fat. The fat, however, is unsaturated and a much better quality of fat than that which would accompany animal protein.

Soy protein is found in all sorts of foods, but often in minor amounts. And some well-known soy products, such as soy sauce, contain little or no genistein. On the other hand, foods like tofu, soy flour, and tempeh are generally excellent sources of genistein.

To help people develop a taste for soy foods, one of Dr. Barnes's assistants has both created and found soy recipes ranging from banana-nut bread to tempeh chili. For Dr. Barnes' birthday, she brought a delicious chocolate-laced tofu cheesecake to the office. "Really, there's no end to the possibilities," says Dr. Barnes.

Seattle nutritionist Mark Messina, like Dr. Barnes, is a big booster of soy foods and recommends Americans eat one serving (½ cup of tofu or 1 cup of soy milk) daily for the isoflavones, which aren't readily found in other foods. He says studies have shown that just one serving daily is enough to lower cancer risk. But the research shows you have to keep it up—the isoflavones don't hang around the body for more than about a day or so.

a sampler of soy products

There are many ways to add soy to your diet. Here is a basic listing of soy products and their uses.

- Tofu is perhaps one of the best known, and can be stir-fried, baked, deep-fried, and even whipped into pudding. Its neutral flavor makes it ideal for marinating.
- Tempeh is a chewy cake made from soybeans. It can be marinated and grilled or cut into chunks and added to soups, stews, chili, or casseroles.
- Soy milk is lactose-free and can be used in almost any way you use cow's milk.
- Soy flour is made from finely ground, roasted soybeans. It adds a pleasant nutty flavor to baked goods. Substitute soy flour for up to one-quarter of the total flour in many baked-good recipes (those designed specifically for soy flour, of course, may require more). Because soy flour doesn't contain any significant amount of gluten, the elastic substance in wheat flour that gives doughs their springy texture, it's best to limit its use in recipes that call for yeast.
- Look for many other soy products in your grocery store. They include textured vegetable (soy) protein (TVP) (usually used in place of ground meats). Fat free, TVP is cheaper than ground beef, and can be reconstituted in water and used in nearly any recipe that calls for

hamburger. You may be eating it already if you buy frozen, microwaveable sausages or similar foods.

Other soy products include soy beans, soy burgers, and hot dogs. Soy margarine, soy cheeses, soy nuts, and even soy-based ice cream and other frozen desserts are available. (And how many other ice creams are you going to find with fiber content?) There is even lactose-free soy "mozzarella" cheese.

A healthy, cancer-protective hamburger? Well, maybe not as healthy as spinach, kale and other leafy green vegetables, but worlds better than that drive-up burger. Try using extra-lean ground beef mixed fifty-fifty with textured vegetable protein. Use your favorite marinade, then roast it instead of grilling or frying, then top it with lots of onions, tomato, and a leafy green vegetable—try spinach instead of iceberg—and a whole grain roll; or better, have it on a bed of mixed greens and sprouts. You may not be on the absolute ideal end of the cancer health spectrum, but you will have improved the nutrient quality over that fast food burger many times.

10

the health advantages of
a vegetarian diet

If all these vegetables are so good for us, then perhaps there's a good argument to be made for eating nothing but vegetables. As it turns out, there is.

How do vegetarian diets compare to omnivorous diets in terms of cancer risk?

In numerous studies that have sought to compare the health of those eating vegetarian diets with those who eat the conventional western/industrial diet, every one has shown vegetarianism to have considerable benefits. Even in sedentary populations and among smokers, vegetarian diets have shown a real advantage over omnivorous diets not only for cancer protection, but overall health as well.

There are differing degrees of vegetarianism. The strictest is the vegan diet, which includes nothing but foods of plant origin. There is what is known as lacto-ovo-vegetarian diet, which includes eggs and dairy products along with foods of plant origin. And then there is the lacto-ovo-vegetarian diet that also includes fish. All of these have shown markedly to lower incidence of cancer, as well as cardiovascular disease and obesity and its attendant complications. These diets also provide a longer overall

life expectancy. This does not mean, however, that if you are a strict vegetarian, you won't get cancer. As discussed in earlier, anyone is a candidate
for cancer.

Several studies of Seventh-Day Adventists, an evangelical religious
denomination with about two and a half million adherents worldwide, have
shown significantly lower rates of cancer morbidity. About half of Seventh
Day Adventists follow a lacto-ovo vegetarian diet, and virtually all adherents abstain from eating pork. Only a small proportion are vegans. Most
avoid the use of alcohol, coffee, tea, hot condiments, and spices. One study
of the sect looked at cancer rates from the late 1950s to the mid-1960s and
showed that rates of death were about half that of the general population
for cancers commonly related to smoking and alcohol use. Rates for other
cancers (such as stomach, pancreas, colon, breast, and ovary) were about
half to a third less than the general, omnivorous population.

A study of Norwegian Seventh-Day Adventists that looked at cancer
rates from the early 1960s to the mid-1980s showed that for those under the
age of 75, the mortality rate from cancer was about 22 percent less than the
omnivorous general population; after age 75, the rates were about the
same. Dutch Seventh-Day Adventists between the mid-1960s to the late
1970s had about half the mortality rate for all cancers than the general population. Japanese adherents showed about two-thirds lower mortality for
men and about a quarter lower mortality for women than the general population.

In addition to comparing the death rates of cancer to the outside population, studies within the California population of the sect have evaluated
the association of specific cancers with various dietary and lifestyle factors. (Seventh-day Adventists are a useful population for internal comparison because of the wide range of dietary habits. For example, within this
population there are a large number of both vegetarians and nonvegetari-
ans, whereas random samples of most Western populations contain too few
vegetarians for meaningful comparisons.) Within the California Seventh-
Day Adventist population, meat consumption was shown not to be related
to risk of prostate cancer in a 1994 study. Likewise, neither consumption of
animal products nor age of first exposure to a vegetarian lifestyle was significantly associated with risk of breast cancer (which brings in the all-
important aspect of lifestyle). On the other hand, higher consumption of
soy-based products, which are a common staple of vegetarian diets in this

population, was associated with a markedly lower risk of pancreatic cancer.

Other studies of vegetarians have also shown a lower incidence of death from cancers than the overall population. A study 1994 of 6,000 British vegetarians who had been followed for 12 years reported an all-cancer mortality rate of less than half that of the overall population. This study also compared the vegetarians against a meat-eating control group that took into account smoking, body mass, and social class (which means that the study attempted to equalize those factors so that what was being measured was the vegetarianism rather than lifestyle factors). The meat-eating controls included friends or relatives of the vegetarians. In both the omnivores and the vegetarians, smoking rates were low, as was the incidence of obesity. In a comparison that was limited to nonsmokers, the all-cancer mortality rate for the vegetarians was still nearly half that of the omnivores.

In a 1996 study, involving 11,000 British men and women recruited through health foods shops, vegetarian societies, and magazines, researchers found overall cancer mortality rates in men to be about half that of the general population, while the rates of women were about a quarter lower.

An 11-year study of nearly 2,000 self-identified German vegetarians found lower overall cancer mortality rates than the general population. The rates were less than half of the "expected" rate for men and about a quarter less for women.

In all of these studies, the vegetarians came mostly from a high socio-economic group, which would indicate that they were likely well-educated, well-read, concerned about health, and probably didn't work in jobs where they might have been exposed regularly to known carcinogens.

what role can vegetarianism play in stopping cancer before it starts?

A vegetarian diet would seem to have somewhat greater benefits for men than women, given the statistics, but it does show benefits for all. This may be due solely to dietary factors, but it may also indicate a significant difference in lifestyle patterns between men and women.

How does vegetarianism help prevent cancer? The mechanisms of cancer, as always, remain somewhat mysterious, but it seems likely that one of the most significant aspects of how a vegetarian diet influences cancer risk is how foods of plant origin affect hormone levels. In both men and women, hormone profiles may be quite different from those of omnivores. This does not mean, however, that omnivores are getting hormones from the meat they eat (although it may be possible that all of us who eat meat get some insignificant amount of hormones from it). What is more likely is that because they consume a larger portion of their energy from plant-derived foods, vegetarians on the whole also consume a much higher percentage of those beneficial fibers and phytochemicals we've been talking about. The effects of vegetarian diets are likely to be due not only to the exclusion of meat (which may increase the risk of bowel cancer, and perhaps cancers of the pancreas, prostate, kidney, and breast), but also to lower incidence of obesity. Body fat, or the adipose tissue, can operate as the body's storehouse (or hiding place) of fat-soluble toxins as well as of fat-soluble anabolic (growth-promoting) hormones.

Although the statistics seem to indicate that you could move yourself into a much lower risk area of the cancer health spectrum by choosing a strictly vegetarian diet, it isn't a necessary step. The key message that comes out of these studies is that the more vegetables and fruits you consume in your diet, the more you will gain in overall better health and lowered cancer risk. That does not have to mean a strict vegetarian diet. Most studies find no additional reduction in cancer risk between vegetarian diets and those that include small amounts of meat (3 ounces or less per day). But the bottom line clearly is to focus your diet on plant-based foods, eating as many vegetables, fruits, and whole grains as possible.

11

the AICR panel's recommendations

Throughout this book, we have made recommendations on various ways you can, through lifestyle and nutritional means, stop cancer before it starts. This chapter is intended to serve as a comprehensive breakdown of those recommendations. If, after reading the book, you want to refer to specific guidelines, this is where to find them.

lifestyle recommendations

1. Nutritional choices. Choose a diet that is predominantly plant-based, rich in a variety of vegetables and fruits, pulses (seeds, peas) or legumes (dried beans) and minimally processed starchy staple foods.

2. Body weight. Avoid being overweight (an increasing problem throughout the population) or underweight (mostly a problem in senior citizens). Limit weight gain during adulthood (for women, after age 18; for men, after age 21) to less than 5 kg (11 pounds).

3. Physical activity. Be active. If all of the benefits of exercise could be

combined in pill form, people would flock to this miracle drug. If your occu-pational activity is low or moderate, take an hour's brisk walk or engage in a similar activity each day. Try to engage in vigorous physical activity (work up a sweat) for a total of at least an hour each week.

dietary and nutritional recommendations

1. Fruits and vegetables. Eat 15 to 30 ounces of a variety of fruits and veg-etables daily year round, or approximately 1 to 2 pounds. If that seems like a lot, it really isn't. Fruits and vegetables are mostly water, and water is heavy. A good-sized apple or pear or orange can often weigh in at close to half a pound. If you have 2 to 3 servings of fruits per day, and 4 to 6 servings of vegetables per day, you're already there.

In terms of proportion of vegetables and fruits, you should eat about 11 to 18 ounces of vegetables, or more than half of your vegetables and fruits intake. Leafy, green vegetables should be a significant part of your total veg-etable intake. You should also remember that eating a variety of these foods is crucial to the mix of nutrients and phytochemicals they supply.

2. Other plant foods. Eat 20 to 30 ounces, or 1½ to 2 pounds daily, or more than 7 servings of a variety of the following energy foods:

- cereals, avoiding those that are highly processed
- pulses or legumes (dried beans and peas)
- roots, tubers, and plantains.

Choose minimally processed foods over highly processed foods, and limit intake of refined sugars—including even supposedly "healthy" sugars such as honey.

3. Alcoholic drinks. Alcohol is an addictive drug that interferes with the metabolism of certain nutrients, and is a class 1 carcinogen, as well as a known cancer promoter. Generally, the more people drink, the poorer and less nutrient-dense their diet will be.

There is no evidence that alcohol reduces the risk of any cancer at any level of intake (despite claims of the antioxidant properties of red wines), and research on breast cancer suggests that women should, if they can, avoid drinking alcohol entirely. There is, however, some evidence that very modest alcohol intake protects men, and perhaps women as well, against coronary heart disease.

The evidence is clear that if you can avoid alcohol entirely, doing so will markedly improve your cancer protection. If you are a woman who has *any* increased risk factor for breast cancer, you should avoid alcohol entirely. If you must drink, the upper limit should be one drink a day for women and two drinks a day for men (a drink is defined as 250 ml [one small glass] of beer, 100 ml of wine, or 25 ml of liquor/spirits). This should provide any available protection against cardiovascular disease (although such protection is available by other means: grapes and grape juice, for example), with only a modest increase in risk for breast cancer.

4. Meat (domesticated red meat: beef, pork, and lamb). The evidence available suggests that if at all possible, it is best to avoid eating red meat; get your protein from other sources, particularly fish, vegetable products (legumes, etc.), skinless poultry, and non-domesticated game animals or birds. Red meat tends to have a much higher concentration of saturated fat—which is, in fact, what often makes it taste so good. Saturated fats are associated with a higher risk of cancer across the board, as well as increased risk of obesity and overweight, also associated with higher cancer risk. If you eat it at all, try to limit red meat intake to no more than 10 percent of your daily energy supply. At an average 2,000 calorie per day energy intake per day, this works out to a limit of about 3 ounces per day. Avoiding processed meats, which can have considerable added salt, sugar, nitrates and other chemicals, is advisable.

5. Fats and oils. Limit consumption of fatty foods, particularly those of animal origin. Choose modest amounts of vegetable oils. These should be predominantly monounsaturated with minimum hydrogenation. Olive oil is an example.

processing recommendations

1. Salt and salting. Limit consumption of salted foods and use of cooking and table salt. Use herbs and spices to season foods.

2. Storage. Do not eat foods liable to fungal contamination. This is particularly true of foods left at room temperature for long periods, particularly during the summer months. Do not eat foods if they become moldy.

Remember the old rule of thumb: When in doubt, throw it out.

3. Preservation. Use refrigeration and other appropriate methods to preserve perishable foods.

4. Additives and residues. When levels of additives, contaminants, or other residues are properly regulated and regulations are observed, their presence in food and drink is almost certainly harmless. However, unregulated or improper use of pesticides and other agricultural chemicals can be a hazard, particularly if the foods come from developing countries. When washing fruits and vegetables, for example, sprayed water is more effective at removing any residue than still water.

5. Preparation. Avoid eating charred food and avoid burning of meat juices. For meat and fish eaters, if you consume meat and fish broiled or grilled in direct flame, or cured and smoked meats, do so only occasionally. Foods that are cooked by steaming, boiling, poaching, stewing, braising, baking, microwaving, or roasting should be the preferred methods of food preparation.

recommendations on dietary supplements

For those who follow the preceding recommendations, dietary supplements are probably unnecessary (unless you have a condition or use a medication that actively depletes a particular nutrient) to achieve the goal of lower cancer risk. Use of dietary supplements instead of a sensible diet can increase cancer risk.

recommendations on tobacco

Avoid it completely.

part IV

recipes and menus

12

recipes for a healthier you

It's sad but true, and perhaps not surprising, that most of us tend to be creatures of habit. While we sometimes find new experiences interesting and exciting, most of us have enough daily stress and frustration in our lives that we don't wish to invite more by trying something new.

But as we hope has been made clear throughout this book, "something new", when it comes to the foods you choose, can often mean making a very large and significant difference in the overall health balance of your life. Following are recipe and menu sections that will indeed suggest trying something new, but that can also reduce much of the hesitation and stress that goes with such new adventures.

In fact, adventure is a good word to describe the process of adding new foods and recipes to your menu. As pointed out in earlier chapters, almost all of us view foods as much more than simply the means of acquiring the energy we need to stay alive. We enjoy the tastes and the experiences they offer. We savor the social side of meals. And for many of us, even the "work" of preparing an interesting meal is really a lot more pleasure than work. All we're suggesting is that you try adding at least a small sense of adventure

225

to the food experience by occasionally experimenting with new tastes, flavors, and textures.

In the recipes that follow, you'll find a combination of approaches to providing foods that are both delicious and good for you. Some of the recipes feature foods with which you are probably quite familiar, perhaps even family favorites. For many of these we've tried to present new ways of preparing or using these foods in order to add more nutrition and health benefits to your meals.

You'll also find that some of the recipes and menu suggestions focus on foods that perhaps are not a regular choice for you or your family, or which you have never tried at all before. It's hoped that trying some at least adds more variety and good nutrition to the meals you enjoy.

The real point of these recipes and menus is to encourage healthier foods, different types of foods, and healthier means of preparing foods. The recipes offered here place a heavy emphasis on adding more vegetables, fruits, and grains to the meals you serve. As the preceding chapters on cancer prevention should have made clear, that's advice we can't afford to ignore if better health and lower cancer risk are a priority.

These recipes also encourage adding new foods, again because there is overwhelming evidence that having variety in your diet is another way of adding substantial and meaningful health benefits.

That need for variety should also carry over to the food choices you make when you are not preparing foods from one of these recipes. Again, it can be fun to be a little more adventurous. When eating out, for example, try a new dish or an order of vegetables that you've never had before. When preparing the kids' school lunches, try adding something totally unexpected, maybe fruits like kiwi, papaya, or mango, or some vegetable sticks, like cucumber, sweet red pepper, or zucchini. When picking out a snack for yourself, skip the usual choices once in a while and reach for something that's again just a little different.

Will you enjoy the new tastes? Will your kids welcome a different snack or dessert suggestion? Maybe yes, maybe no. Either response, from your kids, your spouse, or yourself is fine. You don't have to enjoy every new taste. There are no magic foods. The point is to make the effort, to try that little something different, even if only once in a while, and to encourage the idea that adding variety is a good thing and worth doing. It may take time, but the end result can be a diet that offers excitement, good nutrition, and a lot of help in protecting your body against serious health problems.

Yes, making changes, moving away from the old tried and true, even a little bit, does take some extra effort. It can lead to some less than totally successful experiences, but all the benefits are well worth the trouble.

We urge you to try some of these recipes over the next few weeks. We urge you to start thinking about the foods you choose in a new way. Go for the adventure. You'll find that eventually you'll be looking for new tastes and new food ideas simply because it's fun to do. And, oh yes, you may just be a healthier you for the effort.

openers

spicy spinach dip

MAKES 1 CUP, SERVES ABOUT 4, 45 CALORIES, 2 GRAMS OF FAT PER SERVING.

Feta cheese and horseradish add appealing zip to this velvety deep-green dip. Enjoy it on crackers or stuffed into scooped-out little new potatoes— with their skins, please. This delicious combination gives you a pleasurable powerhouse of caratenoids and flavenoids.

    4 lightly packed cups stemmed fresh spinach leaves
    ½ cup (2 ounces) feta cheese, coarsely crumbled
    2 large scallions, white part only, chopped
    ¼ cup fat-free mayonnaise
    2 teaspoons drained, prepared white horseradish
    1 teaspoon fresh lemon juice
    ¼ cup chopped dill
    Salt and freshly ground pepper to taste

1. In a food processor, finely chop the spinach. Add the feta and scallions. Puree until blended.

2. Add the mayonnaise, horseradish, and lemon juice. Process to blend. Add the dill and process 15 seconds. Season the dip to taste with salt and pepper.

Although this dip keeps 2 to 3 days, it loses some of its zing after 24 hours.

OPTIONS: For a dairy- and cholesterol-free dip, use tofu and tofu mayonnaise (found in natural food stores) in place of the cheese, and fat-free mayonnaise.

COOKING FOR TWO: Blend leftover dip with buttermilk. Chill, garnish with diced cucumber, and serve as a cold soup.

broccoli and mustard dip

MAKES 2 CUPS, SERVES ABOUT 8, 44 CALORIES, 2 GRAMS OF FAT PER SERVING.

Scoop up this creamy dip on carrot sticks and strips of red pepper, and you'll consume a couple of servings of veggies without realizing it. Its zingy flavor pleases even broccoli haters, making it a good way to get them to eat this cruciferous powerhouse of healthful nutrients.

If you do not eat dairy, use 8 ounces of soft tofu in place of the cheese and buttermilk.

    4 cups (about 8 ounces) broccoli florets
    ½ cup reduced-fat ricotta cheese
    ¼ cup Dijon mustard
    2 cloves roasted garlic
    ¼ cup low-fat buttermilk
    Salt and freshly ground pepper to taste

1. In a large pot of boiling water, cook the broccoli 5 minutes, until tender but not soft. With a slotted spoon, remove and immediately plunge into a bowl of ice water. When the broccoli is completely cooled, drain well and place in the bowl of a food processor.

2. Puree the broccoli. Add the ricotta, mustard, garlic, and buttermilk. Process until well blended. Season to taste with salt and pepper. Pour the dip into a serving bowl or plastic container. Cover and refrigerate to let the flavors develop, from 1 hour to overnight, before serving. Serve with carrot and celery sticks, and strips of red pepper.

Tightly covered, this dip keeps in the refrigerator for 2 to 3 days.

OPTIONS: Use a 10-ounce package of frozen spinach, defrosted and squeezed dry, instead of the broccoli.

COOKING FOR TWO: If you have leftover dip after entertaining, mash it with boiled potatoes or use it as a sauce over baked or poached chicken breast.

roasted garlic

MAKES 1 HEAD, SERVES ABOUT 2, 23 CALORIES, LESS THAN 1 GRAM OF FAT PER SERVING.

Always keep roasted garlic on hand to add to a variety of foods. Roasting garlic brings out its flavor in a gentler way than sautéing. It is so easy to make that you can throw a head or two of garlic into the oven anytime you are making something else. Mashed into potatoes, soups, and salad dressings, you'll find that roasted garlic adds creamy texture as well as flavor and beneficial phytochemicals.

    1 large (or 2 small) head garlic,
    ¼ teaspoon olive oil

1. Preheat the oven to 375°F. (You can also use a toaster oven.)

2. Cut the garlic horizontally across the top so most or all of the cloves are exposed. Rub the garlic with the oil, using your hands.

3. Wrap the garlic in foil. Bake until soft and lightly browned, 45 to 60 minutes.

Roasted garlic keeps in the refrigerator, wrapped in foil for 4 to 5 days.

carrot and red lentil pâté

MAKES 2 CUPS, SERVES ABOUT 10, 64 CALORIES, 2 GRAMS OF FAT PER SERVING.

Serve this colorful spread, warmed with the flavors of orange and rosemary, as an hors d'oeuvre or light opener for a meal. Red lentils cook down to a velvety puree in just 20 minutes. They are rich in fiber, which is essential for good health and something most of us find hard to get in the recommended quantity each day.

    2 teaspoons extra-virgin olive oil
    2 medium carrots, cut in ¾-inch slices
    1 small onion, chopped

1 clove garlic, chopped
½ cup red lentils, rinsed and drained
2 strips orange zest, each 2 inches x ½ inch
Juice of 1 orange, about ½ cup
1½ teaspoons chopped fresh rosemary, or ¾ teaspoon dried, crushed
1½ cups vegetable broth or water
4 ounces soft tofu
Salt and freshly ground pepper to taste

1. Heat the oil in a large saucepan over medium-high heat. Sauté the carrots, onion, and garlic until the onion is translucent, about 5 minutes.

2. Add the lentils, orange zest, orange juice, rosemary, and broth or water. Bring just to a boil, cover, reduce the heat, and simmer until the carrots are soft and the lentils are mushy, about 20 minutes.

3. Transfer the cooked lentils and carrots, with the orange zest and any cooking liquid, to the bowl of a food processor. Puree the mixture. Crumble in the tofu and process until completely blended. Season to taste with salt and pepper.

4. Pack the pâté into a serving bowl and cool almost to room temperature. Cover with plastic wrap and refrigerate until ready to serve. This pâté can be made 2 to 3 days before serving.

OPTIONS: This puree is good to serve warm, along with rice and a green vegetable, such as collards or broccoli, as a meatless dinner.

COOKING FOR TWO: First, enjoy scoops of this pâté on a bed of romaine lettuce. In a day or two, serve the rest stuffed into celery sticks.

soups

chicken and rice soup with mushroom "croutons"

SERVES 4, 178 CALORIES, 5 GRAMS OF FAT PER SERVING.

Chicken and rice soup is old-fashioned comfort food. In this up dated version, brown and wild rices add fiber and flair. Mushroom "croutons" are an original touch which adds cancer-preventing terpines, along with rich flavor. For a light supper, serve with a green salad and Cinnamon-Raisin Bread Pudding (page 307).

2 teaspoons canola oil
2 cups coarsely diced mushrooms
4 cups rich, de fatted chicken broth
¼ cup finely chopped onion
1 small carrot, thinly sliced
1 small rib celery, thinly sliced
1 cup diced cooked chicken breast
½ cup cooked brown rice
½ cup cooked wild rice
Salt and freshly ground pepper to taste

1. In a medium non stick skillet, heat the oil over medium-high heat. Sauté the mushrooms until they give up their liquid, about 6 minutes. Raise the heat and cook the mushrooms, stirring often, until they are browned and slightly dry, about 12 minutes. Set aside.

2. In a large, deep saucepan, use ¼ cup of the broth in place of oil to sauté the onion, carrots, and celery over medium-high heat for 1 minute. Reduce the heat, cover tightly, and cook gently until the vegetables are not quite tender, about 7 minutes.

3. Add the rest of the chicken broth, the cooked chicken, and brown and wild rices. Cook until they are heated through.

4. To serve, divide the soup among 4 soup bowls. Garnish each with the mushroom "croutons."

OPTIONS: Use chicken meatballs as in Escarole Soup with Meatballs (page 237) in place of cooked chicken. Garnish with a chopped scallion or some dill.

COOKING FOR TWO: Add a diced cooked potato or cooked lentils to the leftovers and serve as a main dish stew.

greek chickpea soup

SERVES 4, 193 CALORIES, 3 GRAMS OF FAT PER SERVING.

Greek cooking is often alluring in its simplicity. Here, the cooking liquid from diced chickpeas is the base for a fat-free flavorful soup embellished with vibrant green ribbons of tangy arugula. Lemon juice adds a refreshing, unexpected note.

- 1 cup dried chickpeas
- ½ cup chopped onion
- 1 whole garlic clove, peeled
- 1 tablespoon lemon juice
- 1 cup arugula, cut in ½-inch ribbons
- Salt and freshly ground pepper to taste

1. In a small Dutch oven or heavy pot, combine the dried chickpeas with 6 cups cold water. Bring to a boil. Reduce the heat and simmer, covered, for 30 minutes. Add the onions and garlic, and continue cooking, covered, until the chickpeas are quite soft, up to 2 hours.

2. In a food processor or blender, process 1 cup of the cooked chickpeas with ½ cup of the soup liquid and the garlic clove, until some of the chickpeas are pureed but some remain coarsely chopped. Mix this back into the pot. Stir in the lemon juice.

3. Season the soup to taste with salt and freshly ground pepper and ladle into serving bowls. Mix ¼ of the thin arugula ribbons into each bowl just until the greens are wilted. Serve immediately.

kale and white bean soup

SERVES 4, 311 CALORIES, 4 GRAMS OF FAT PER SERVING.

The Portuguese call this soup Caldo Verde. They add sausage to give it smoky flavor. In this meatless version, parsnip and Rich Vegetable Stock (page 240) give an equally satisfying character to this hearty soup. Kale is a leafy green rich in calcium and beta-carotene. Here is a great way to enjoy it. Serve this stew like soup accompanied by toasted slices of Whole Wheat Bread with Fresh Herbs (page 282) for a light meal.

2   teaspoons extra-virgin olive oil
2   cups chopped onion
1   small parsnip, peeled and chopped
2   cloves garlic
3   cups Rich Vegetable Stock or canned broth
3   cups kale, stemmed and cut crosswise into ½-inch strips
1   medium red-skinned potato, peeled and cut in ¾-inch cubes
⅛   teaspoon red pepper flakes
15-ounce can cannelini beans, rinsed and drained
Salt and freshly ground pepper to taste

1. In a small Dutch oven, heat the oil over medium-high heat. Add the onion, parsnip, and garlic. Sauté until the onion is translucent, about 6 minutes. Add the stock or broth, kale, potato and pepper flakes. Bring the soup to boil, reduce the heat, and simmer 20 minutes, until the kale is tender.

2. Add the beans and simmer until they are heated through.

OPTIONS: Kale, beans, potatoes and corn go together well. Try this soup using 1 cup of corn kernels, and omitting the parsnip.

COOKING FOR TWO: This soup freezes nicely, so pour what you do not want to eat into portion-size containers and save it for a meal when you don't want to cook.

kidney bean and quinoa chowder

SERVES 4, 273 CALORIES, 6 GRAMS OF FAT PER SERVING.

We think of corn as a vegetable, but, like quinoa, it is also a grain. Here, they are paired to add sweetness, color, and fiber to a light but hearty soup. This stew like chowder calls for a richly flavored broth, like Rich Vegetable Stock (page 240), but several canned ones on the market will do nicely if you don't have this on hand.

2   teaspoons olive oil
¾   cup chopped onion
1   rib celery, cut in ½-inch slices
¼   cup quinoa, well rinsed and drained
1   small zucchini, cut in ½-inch cubes
1   medium red or white potato, cut in ½-inch cubes
½   Granny Smith or Fuji apple, peeled and cored, cut in ½-inch cubes
6   cups vegetable broth
10-ounce can kidney beans, drained and rinsed
1   cup frozen, canned, or fresh corn kernels
Salt and freshly ground pepperto taste
2   tablespoons chopped fresh cilantro, for garnish

1. Heat the oil in a large saucepan over medium-high heat. Sauté the onion and celery until the onion is translucent, about 5 minutes.

2. Add the quinoa, zucchini, potato, and apple. Pour in the broth. Bring to a boil, reduce the heat, and simmer until the potatoes are tender and the grain is cooked, about 15 minutes.

3. Add the beans and corn. Cook until they are heated through. Season the chowder to taste with salt and pepper. Ladle into warm bowls, garnish with the cilantro, and serve.

OPTIONS: Along with the beans and corn, add 1 to 2 corn tortillas, torn into bite-size pieces, or ¾ cup cubed cooked chicken.

COOKING FOR TWO: This soup keeps 2 to 3 days and reheats nicely. So take a break, then serve it again in a couple of days. The second time, garnish with a squirt of fresh lime juice instead of the cilantro.

french onion soup

SERVES 6, 264 CALORIES, 6 GRAMS OF FAT PER SERVING.

Onion soup usually requires a rich beef broth. This recipe calls instead for chicken stock. Using a homemade stock like Rich Chicken Stock (see page 239) really makes a difference, especially in sodium. It need not be a very rich broth. In fact, a mediumly intense one is better because it lets the onions' flavor shine through. An abundance of onions, stewed in their own juices and then well-browned, makes this a particularly hearty onion soup, especially if you include a slice of cheese-topped bread.

    4 pounds (3to 5) large Spanish onions
    1 tablespoon-extra virgin olive oil
    1 tablespoon Dijon mustard
    Salt and freshly ground pepper to taste
    ¾ teaspoon dried thyme
    4 cups chicken stock or defatted low-sodium broth
    6 slices whole wheat or white Italian or French bread
    6 tablespoons shredded low-fat Swiss cheese

1. Cut the onions in half. Cut the halves cross wise into ⅜-inch dices.

2. In a Dutch oven, heat the oil over medium-high heat. Add the onions, stirring them with a wooden spoon until they are separated and coated with the oil. Cook the onions, stirring occasionally, until they are limp, about 10 minutes.

3. Cover the pot and let the onions steam in their own juices for 10 minutes, reducing the heat so the onions do not color.

4. Uncover the pot. Keep cooking the onions, stirring occasionally, until they are golden brown, about 15 minutes. Mix in the mustard and thyme.

5. Add the chicken broth and bring the soup to barely a boil. Simmer for 20 minutes. Add salt and pepper, if needed. If possible, let the soup cool, and reheat before serving.

6. Toast the bread or let it sit out overnight to get hard.

7. Heat the soup. Ladle the soup into heat-proof bowls. Preheat the broiler. Place a slice of the bread on top of each bowl. Sprinkle the cheese to cover the bread. Place each bowl under the broiler to melt the cheese. Serve immediately.

escarole soup with meat balls

SERVES 4, 195 CALORIES, 5 GRAMS OF FAT PER SERVING.

Meatballs and a generous helping of greens make this Italian-inspired soup a light one-dish meal. Using chicken makes the meatballs particularly fine. The carrot adds sweetness that contrasts pleasantly with the slightly bitter flavor of the greens. The rich stock knits all the flavors together nicely.

½ pound (1 cup) ground chicken
¼ cup grated carrot
¼ cup finely chopped onion
1 small clove garlic, minced
½ teaspoon salt
Freshly ground pepper to taste
Pinch cayenne pepper
1 egg white
3 tablespoons bread crumbs
6 cups Rich Chicken Stock (page 243)
1 piece lemon zest, 1 inch x 2 inches
6 cups escarole, cut crosswise in ½-inch strips
1 tablespoon grated Parmesan cheese (optional)

1. For the meatballs: In a medium bowl, combine the chicken with the carrot, onion, garlic, salt, 5 to 6 grinds of the black pepper, and the cayenne, using a fork. Stir in the egg white and bread crumbs. Wetting your hands with cold water, form this mixture into 24 one-inch balls, setting them on a plate as you work. Cover the plate with plastic wrap and refrigerate, from 30 minutes, to overnight.

2. For the soup: In a large, deep saucepan, bring the chicken stock with the lemon zest just to a boil, reduce the heat, and simmer gently for 5 minutes. Mix in the escarole and continue cooking for 5 minutes. Add the chilled meatballs and cook until they are firm and no pink shows in the center, 6 to 8 minutes. Remove the lemon zest. Ladle the soup with the meatballs into individual bowls and serve, sprinkled with the cheese, if using.

OPTIONS: In place of escarole, use Swiss chard cut into strips; the cooking time remains the same. Do not use ground turkey; it will make dry, hard meatballs.

COOKING FOR TWO: Form half the meat into balls, and half into two patties. Pan-cook the patties and serve as burgers the next day. Add cooked rice or a diced new potato to half the soup, to serve with the burgers.

ten-minute gazpacho

SERVES 4, 65 CALORIES, 3 GRAMS OF FAT PER SERVING.

Chilled gazpacho is one of the most refreshing things you can serve on a hot day. Adding to its appeal, no cooking is required. Start with a top-quality tomato juice, and use a trick—replace the traditionally used stale bread with bread crumbs to thicken the soup, and you'll be out of the kitchen in a wink. And tasting this lycopene-laden, vibrant soup, no one will be any the wiser.

    2 cups tomato juice
    2 garlic cloves, chopped
    2 teaspoons olive oil
    2 tablespoons bread crumbs
    1 tablespoon white wine vinegar
    Salt and freshly grounded pepper to taste
    ¼ cup seeded and diced cucumber
    ¼ cup finely diced green bell pepper
    1 plum tomato, seeded and finely diced
    ¼ cup red onion, finely diced
    ¼ cup zucchini, finely diced (optional)
    1 hard-boiled egg white, finely chopped (optional)

1. Place the tomato juice, garlic, and olive oil in a blender and process until the garlic is pureed. Add the bread crumbs and vinegar, and blend to combine. Season to taste with salt and pepper. Pour into a covered container and chill well, from 2 hours to overnight.

2. Check the seasoning and adjust, if necessary. Divide the soup among 4 serving bowls. Add 1 tablespoon each of the diced cucumber, pepper, tomato, and onion, plus the zucchini and egg white, if using.

rich chicken stock

MAKES 2 QUARTS, SERVES ABOUT 6, 20 CALORIES, LESS THAN 1
GRAM OF FAT PER SERVING.

A good stock adds intensity to dishes while staying in the background.
Chicken wings make a particularly flavorful stock. Cooling the stock with
the solids in it lets you extract the maximum flavor from them. A generous
amount of onions adds sweetness. If you like more assertive flavors in a
broth, feel free to add more vegetables, herbs, or whatever pleases you.

    2 pounds chicken wings
    1 cup coarsely chopped onion
    1 large carrot, cut in 2-inch pieces
    1 rib celery, cut in 2-inch pieces
    1 small parsnip
    6 sprigs parsley
    1 teaspoon peppercorns

1. Place the chicken, onion, carrot, celery, parsnip, parsley, and peppercorns in a stockpot or pasta pot. Add 12 cups cold water. Bring the liquid to
just below a boil and hold it where bubbles rise gently to the surface. Skim
off any scum that accumulates. Cook for 2 hours, until the liquid is reduced
by almost one-third.

2. Let the stock cool in the pot until it is lukewarm. Pour carefully through a
strainer into quart containers. Save the chicken wings. Cover and refrigerate the stock overnight. Skim off all the fat that accumulates and solidifies
on the surface.

3. Pick over the chicken wings while they are still warm, separating the bits
of meat from the skin and bones. Reserve this meat to use in soup or for a
chicken salad.

rich vegetable stock

MAKES 3 QUARTS, SERVES ABOUT 9, 27 CALORIES, LESS THAN 1 GRAM OF FAT PER SERVING.

This intense broth adds interest to cooked grains and contributes depth of flavor to soups. Though complex, the flavors in this stock blend well in all kinds of meatless dishes. Most of the instant and canned vegetable broth you can buy is loaded with sodium. It may also contain other undesirable ingredients such as sugar, MSG, and various additives. Remember to freeze some of this homemade stock as ice cubes so you can use small amounts for steaming zucchini, spinach, and other vegetables.

- 1 medium leek, white part only, chopped
- 1 medium onion, halved
- 3 cups (4 to 5 leaves) torn romaine lettuce
- 2 cups coarsely chopped green cabbage
- 1½ cups chopped carrot
- 1 cup chopped zucchini
- ¾ cup stemmed green beans, halved
- 3 ribs celery, cut in 4 pieces each
- ½ cup quartered mushrooms
- ¼ cup chopped celery leaves
- 15 stems parsley
- 1½ cups canned whole tomatoes, with 1 cup of their liquid
- 2 bay leaves
- ½ teaspoon dried thyme
- ¼ teaspoon whole peppercorns

1. In a large stock pot or pasta pot, place the leek, onion, lettuce, cabbage, carrot, zucchini, green beans, celery, mushrooms, celery leaves, and parsley stems. Add 12 cups cold water. Bring to a boil and simmer 30 minutes.

2. Add the tomatoes and juice, bay leaves, thyme, and peppercorns. Simmer for 30 minutes. Let the stock cool with the vegetables and seasoning. Strain and refrigerate or freeze.

main dishes

chicken breast with red pepper sauce

SERVES 4, 184 CALORIES, 6 GRAMS OF FAT PER SERVING.

This dish is so simple to make that you can enjoy it any night, though its brilliant color and flavor makes it a good choice for special occasions. Both the sauce and the chicken are good served either warm or at room temperature. The red peppers are rich in vitamin C and beta-carotene, while the garlic provides the goodness found in alliums. But the Mediterranean exuberance of this dish is what makes it so appealing.

2   medium red bell peppers
1   pound boneless chicken breast, well-trimmed, cut in 4 pieces
1   teaspoon olive oil
1   teaspoon chopped fresh rosemary, or ½ teaspoon dried, crushed
1   tablespoon extra-virgin olive oil
4   cloves roasted garlic
1   teaspoon balsamic vinegar
Salt and freshly ground pepper to taste
4   sprigs fresh rosemary, for garnish (optional)

1. Preheat the oven to 500°F.

2. Place the peppers on a baking sheet covered with foil. Roast for 30 minutes, until the skin feels loose to the touch. The peppers will still be somewhat firm. Place the peppers in a paper bag and close tightly. Let the peppers sit 15 to 20 minutes.

3. With your fingers, pull the skin from the peppers, holding them over a bowl to catch the pieces. Halve the peppers, remove the stems, seeds, and ribs. Set aside.

4. Coat each piece of chicken with ¼ teaspoon of the oil. Sprinkle each with ¼ teaspoon of the rosemary.

5. Heat a medium, heavy, non-stick skillet over medium-high heat. Cook the chicken until it is lightly browned and just firm to the touch, about 5 minutes on each side. When pierced with a knife, juices from the chicken should run clear. Transfer the cooked chicken to a plate.

6. Make the sauce: Puree the peppers in a blender. Add the remaining olive oil, garlic, and vinegar and blend until sauce is fluffy and just slightly "grainy." Season to taste with salt and pepper.

7. Pour a generous amount of the sauce on each of four dinner plates. Cut each chicken fillet crosswise into four pieces. Arrange the pieces of chicken on the sauce in a pinwheel, laying them cut-side down. Garnish with a sprig of rosemary in the center of the pinwheel and serve.

OPTIONS: The chicken can be poached in chicken broth, or steamed.

Serve the sauce with baked sole, flounder, or halibut. It also goes well with baked eggplant.

COOKING FOR TWO: Use one chicken breast.

baked tandoori chicken

SERVES 4, 258 CALORIES, 10 GRAMS OF FAT PER SERVING.

Tandoori chicken is always a favorite, but firing up the grill to make it is not always convenient. Here, baking provides the way to enjoy this succulent dish anytime. Using the oven is also a more healthful way of cooking than charring the meat on the grill, and it brings out the flavor of the spices. In fact, this aromatically seasoned chicken is excellent in salads—make extra for leftovers.

    1 cup fat-free yogurt
    1 small onion, coarsely chopped
    4 garlic cloves
    1½ piece gingerroot, peeled and coarsely chopped
    2 teaspoons ground coriander
    1 teaspoon ground cumin

½ teaspoon turmeric
¼ teaspoon ground cinnamon
¼ teaspoon ground clove
¼ teaspoon ground mace
¼ teaspoon grated nutmeg
2 tablespoons vegetable oil
Juice of ½ lemon (2 to 3 tablespoons)
2 whole chicken breasts, split and skinned

1. Preheat the oven to 375°F. In a blender or food processor, combine the yogurt, onion, garlic, and ginger, and puree together. Add the coriander, cumin, turmeric, cinnamon, cloves, mace, nutmeg, oil, and lemon juice, and blend.

2. Cut 2 slits in each piece of chicken, slashing it along the grain to make a slit 2 to 3 inches long and almost but not completely into the bone. Place the chicken in a plastic bag or a glass, stainless steel, or plastic container large enough to hold the pieces in one layer. Pour the yogurt mixture over the chicken and rub to be sure it coats the meat on all sides. Marinate the chicken in the refrigerator one hour to overnight.

3. Arrange the chicken in one layer in a shallow baking dish. Bake until the pieces run clear when a breast is pierced with a knife at its thickest point and no pink shows in the center, 35 to 45 minutes, depending on the size of the breasts. Serve, accompanied by cooked basmati rice and a green salad.

OPTIONS: Let the chicken cool and use to make an Indian chicken salad, with green peas, mango, scallions, and cooked rice in a yogurt dressing with chutney.

COOKING FOR TWO: Halve the recipe, or use the leftover chicken to make a salad, served cold, or add to soup.

turkey cutlets in honey-mustard sauce

SERVES 4, 201 CALORIES, 2 GRAMS OF FAT PER SERVING.

When time is short but you want a substantial, relaxing dinner, this is a perfect dish. While it simmers, toss some broccoli in the microwave, quick-cook some rice, and you can sit down to a most civilized meal in well under 30 minutes. It's a well-balanced one, too.

    4 4-ounce turkey cutlets
    ⅓ cup flour
    1 cup buttermilk
    3 tablespoons Dijon mustard
    2 teaspoons honey
    Salt and freshly ground pepper to taste

1. Coat the cutlets with the flour.

2. Generously spray a medium, nonstick skillet with cooking spray. Add the cutlets to the pan and set it over medium-high heat. When the cutlets are lightly colored on the bottom, turn and brown the top.

3. Add the buttermilk to the pan. Mix in the mustard and honey, salt and pepper. Simmer, reducing the heat if necessary, until the cutlets are cooked through, about 10 minutes. No pink should show in the center if you cut into a cutlet. Serve immediately, with the sauce spooned over the cutlets.

OPTIONS: Use chicken cutlets. Add a ½ teaspoon dried basil along with the mustard, or use a tarragon mustard.

COOKING FOR TWO: Use half the amount of each ingredient. If the liquid cooks out too quickly, add 1 to 2 tablespoons chicken broth.

venison with cranberries and juniper

SERVES 4, 374 CALORIES, 11 GRAMS OF FAT PER SERVING.

Lean cuts of venison, such as the loin, have about half the fat and a third of the calories of lean beef, according to studies by the U.S. Department of Agriculture. It also has a fine grain. Most of the venison available today is farmed, and much of this is sold frozen. It has a relatively mild taste, though it certainly is more assertive than that of beef. Because venison loin is so lean, it needs marinating and careful cooking so it stays pink and does not dry out. Usually, red wine is used when cooking venison, but the acid in cranberry juice works nicely, too. Serve with potato gratin and braised red cabbage.

- 1 tablepoon olive oil
- ¼ cup carrots, chopped
- ¼ cup onion, chopped
- 1 tablespoon shallot, chopped
- 1 garlic clove, chopped
- 1½ cups unfiltered apple juice
- ½ cup defrosted cranberry juice concentrate
- ¼ cup red wine vinegar
- 2 parsley sprigs
- 1 bay leaf
- 1½ teaspoons crushed juniper berries
- ½ teaspoon salt
- ½ teaspoon freshly ground pepper
- ¾ cup beef broth
- 1 teaspoon chopped tarragon, or ½ teaspoon dried
- 4 venison medallions cut from the loin, 4 ounces each
- 1 tablespoon plus 1 teaspoon unsalted butter
- ¾ cup beef broth
- 1 teaspoon chopped tarragon, or ½ teaspoon dried
- ¼ cup pomegranate seeds, or 2 tablespoons dried cranberries, plumped in apple juice for 15 minutes, for garnish

1. For the marinade: Heat 2 teaspoons of the oil in a medium saucepan over medium-high heat. Sauté the carrots, onion, shallot, and garlic until brown,

6 to 7 minutes, stirring often. Add the apple and cranberry juice concentrate, vinegar, parsley, bay leaf, juniper, salt, and pepper. Bring the marinade to a boil, reduce heat, and simmer for 10 minutes. Cool completely.

2. Arrange the venison in a glass dish, plastic box with tight-fitting cover, or a heavy plastic bag with tight closure. Add the marinade and place in the refrigerator, from 6 hours to overnight.

3. For the sauce: Remove the meat from the marinade and set aside, covered lightly with plastic wrap to keep it from drying out. Remove the parsley and bay leaf from the marinade. Pour the marinade into a medium, nonreactive saucepan. Bring to a boil over medium-high heat and cook until the liquid is reduced to 1 cup. Add the beef broth and tarragon and boil to reduce back to 1 cup. Set aside.

4. To cook the meat, heat 1 teaspoon butter with 1 teaspoon olive oil in a medium skillet over medium-high heat. Pat the venison with a paper towel to make sure it is dry. Cook until browned, about 5 minutes, then turn and brown on the second side, 4 to 5 minutes longer. The venison should be pink in the center. Set the venision on a plate and pour the sauce from the saucepan into the skillet. With a wooden spoon, scrape any browned bits into the liquid.

5. Carefully pour the hot liquid and the solids into the container of a blender. Process until the solids are pureed into the liquid. Cut the butter into 4 pieces and whirl in the blender with the sauce. Adjust the seasoning to taste with salt and pepper. Pour some of the sauce on individual plates. Place a venison medallion on each plate. Garnish with the pomegranate seeds or drained, plumped cranberries and serve.

OPTIONS: If you like, leave the venison in one piece. Marinate and roast it in a 350°F. oven until an instant-read thermometer placed in the venison registers 130 degrees and the meat is pink inside.

COOKING FOR TWO: If the butcher can provide just 2 medallions, go for it. Use the entire recipe amounts for the marinade and sauce. Keep the sauce to use with pork or lamb.

confetti meatloaf

SERVES 6, 218 CALORIES, 4 GRAMS OF FAT PER SERVING.

Mashed potatoes replace the usual bread crumbs as the binder in this meatloaf. Studded colorfully with vegetables, it has the satisfying quality of meatloaf made with red meat, but is lower in fat. Serve it hot, or chill and slice it for sandwiches.

- 1 teaspoon olive oil
- 1 small leek, white part only, chopped
- ½ cup finely diced carrots
- ½ cup chopped onion
- 1 pound ground turkey
- 1 egg white, beaten until frothy
- ½ cup instant mashed potatoes
- 1 teaspoon dried thyme
- ¼ bouillon cube
- ½ teaspoon salt
- ¼ teaspoon freshly ground pepper
- 1 cup cooked cubed potatoes
- 5 thin slices tomato

1. Preheat the oven to 375°F.

2. In a medium, nonstick skillet, heat the oil over medium-high heat. Sauté the leeks, carrots, and onions for 2 to 3 minutes, until the leeks start to soften. Cover the pan, reduce the heat, and let the vegetables cook in their own juices for 8 minutes, taking care not to let them brown. When the carrots are *al dente,* uncover the pan, remove it from the heat, and set aside to cool for 10 minutes. (This work can be done up to 8 hours ahead and the vegetables refrigerated in a closed container.)

3. In a large bowl, combine the turkey with the cooked vegetables, egg white, instant mashed potatoes, and thyme, mixing them with a fork until evenly blended.

4. In a small cup, dissolve the bouillon in 1 tablespoon hot water. Mix this into the meat, together with the salt and freshly ground pepper. Mix in the cubed potatoes.

5. Pack the meatloaf firmly into a 9-inch x 5-inch x 3-inch loaf pan. Arrange the tomato slices over the top of the meat, overlapping them slightly. Wrap the meatloaf in aluminum foil and bake for 45 minutes. Unwrap and bake 15 to 20 minutes longer, until the juices run clear when the meatloaf is pierced with a knife or the internal temperature registers 165°F on an instant-read thermometer. Let sit 20 minutes before slicing.

bronzed pork medallions

SERVES 4, 160 CALORIES, 4 GRAMS OF FAT PER SERVING.

Pork and fruit go so well together. These pan-cooked medallions, simmered in a blend of fruit juice and herbs, prove there is room for everything you like in a healthful, varied diet. Take care in cooking them, as this lean cut of meat dries out quickly if overdone. Serve with Braised Red Cabbage (page 287).

    1   tablespoon dark brown sugar
    1   teaspoon chili powder
    1   teaspoon paprika, sweet or hot
    ½   teaspoon dried oregano
    4   pork medallions, well-trimmed, each 3 to 4 ounces
    ¼   cup apple cider or juice
    2   tablespoons orange juice
    1   teaspoon Worcestershire sauce
    Salt and freshly ground pepper to taste

1. In a small bowl, combine the sugar, chili powder, paprika, and oregano. Rub ¼ teaspoon of this mixture into each side of the pork medallions. Arrange the meat on a plate, cover with plastic wrap, and let sit for 15 minutes at room temperature.

2. Generously spray a nonstick skillet with cooking spray. Over high heat, sear the meat on both sides. Add the apple cider or juice, orange juice, and Worcestershire sauce to the pan and immediately reduce the heat. Simmer until no pink shows when you cut into the meat, about 10 minutes, turning the meat once. The liquid in the pan should be syrupy. If it is not, remove the meat to a serving plate and boil the juices until thickened. Add salt and pepper if needed. Spoon the sauce over the meat and serve.

OPTIONS: Use turkey cutlets in place of the pork. If you like heat, mix a dash of cayenne in the rubbing spices.

COOKING FOR TWO: Halve the amount of each ingredient except the juices and Worcestershire sauce.

picadillo

SERVES 4, 243 CALORIES, 6 GRAMS OF FAT PER SERVING.

Mushrooms and potatoes in this enlightened Picadillo cleverly conceal the fact that it calls for less meat than traditional recipes. Draining the cooked meat well further reduces the amount of fat in this hefty dish. Capers, olives, and cinnamon provide an intrigue of complex flavors. Serve over steamed or boiled rice.

¾ pound lean chopped meat (6 percent fat)
1 cup chopped onion
1½ cups unpeeled red potato, cut in ½-inch cubes
1 cup chopped portobello mushroom
1 teaspooon ground cinnamon
1 teaspoon dried oregano
1 cup canned whole plum tomatoes
3 tablespoons dried currants
2 tablespoons drained capers
2 tablespoons chopped pitted green Spanish olives
Salt and freshly ground pepper to taste

1. In a large, nonstick skillet over medium-high heat, brown the meat, breaking it up with a wooden spoon. Tilt the pan so the fat released in cooking runs to one side. Using a slotted spoon, remove the meat to a plate. Set it aside. Rinse and dry the pan.

2. Set the dry skillet over medium high heat. Sauté the onions, potatoes, and mushrooms until the onions are lightly browned, about 10 minutes, stirring often. Mix in the cinnamon and oregano. Add the tomatoes, breaking them up with the spoon.

3. Add the cooked meat to the pan, along with the currants, capers, and olives. Simmer the Picadillo over medium heat for 5 minutes to blend the flavors. Season to taste with salt and freshly ground pepper. Serve over cooked rice.

southwestern meatloaf with spinach

SERVES 8, 167 CALORIES, 4 GRAMS OF FAT PER SERVING.

Getting grains and a generous amount of vegetables into a meal is sometimes a challenge. Here, oats, spinach, corn, and tomatoes are blended right into the main course, making it easier to reach the five-a-day goal. They also help you stretch the meat to more servings. Everyone loves the bold flavor in this meatloaf, which is equally good served hot or cold.

½ cup rolled oats (not quick cooking or instant)
2 egg whites, beaten until frothy
1 cup tomato, seeded and chopped
1¼ pounds ground turkey
1 tablespoon chili powder
1 teaspoon oregano
½ teaspoon salt
¼ teaspoon freshly ground pepper
1 package defrosted frozen spinach, squeezed dry
½ cup frozen, canned, or fresh corn kernels
¼ cup chili sauce or ketchup

1. Preheat the oven to 375°F.

2. In a large bowl, using a fork, mix together the oats, egg whites, and tomato. Blend in the turkey, chili powder, oregano, salt, and freshly ground pepper. Mix in the spinach and corn.

3. Pack the meatloaf firmly into a 9-inch x 5-inch x 3-inch loaf pan. Bake, uncovered, for 45 minutes. Spread the chili sauce or ketchup over the top and continue baking until the juices of the meat run clear when the meatloaf is pierced with a knife, or the temperature in the center registers 165°F on an instant-read thermometer.

4. Let the meatloaf sit for 15 minutes before slicing, or cool it in the pan.

turkey pot pie

SERVES 4, 415 CALORIES, 7 GRAMS OF FAT PER SERVING.

Topped with mashed potatoes rather than a baked crust, this is really a shepherd's pie. The potatoes are easier to make and add vitamin C, while helping you avoid the fat required for a flaky crust. The vegetables and herbs in this homey dish give big flavor along with good nutrients.

FILLING:
2 teaspoons canola oil
½ cup finely chopped onion
½ cup finely chopped leek, white part only
2 carrots, cut in ½-inch slices
1 small parsnip, cut in ½-inch slices
1 rib celery, cut in ½-inch slices
¾ cup defatted chicken broth
2 large mushrooms, each cut in 8 wedges
8 ounces cooked turkey breast, cut in 1-inch cubes
1 tablespoon flour
1 cup evaporated skim milk
½ teaspoon dried rosemary, or 1 teaspoon fresh
½ teaspoon dried thyme, or 1 teaspoon fresh
Dash hot pepper sauce
½ teaspoon salt
Freshly ground pepper

TOPPING:
1½ pounds yellow- or white-fleshed potatoes, peeled
¼ cup low-fat buttermilk
1 tablespoon Dijon mustard
1 tablespoon extra-virgin olive oil
1 egg white

1. Preheat oven to 350°F.

2. In a medium, nonstick skillet, heat the oil over medium-high heat. Sauté the onions, leeks, carrots, parsnip, and celery until the onions soften, about 8 minutes.

3. Pour in ½ cup of the chicken broth. Cover tightly, reduce the heat to medium, and cook 10 minutes. Add the mushrooms and cook 10 minutes.

4. While the vegetables cook, cut the potatoes for the topping into halves or quarters and boil until easily pierced with a knife, 15 to 20 minutes. Set aside, undrained until the filling is done.

5. Add the turkey to the vegetables. Stir in the flour and cook 1 to 2 minutes, until the flour is well absorbed. Mix in the remaining ¼ cup of chicken broth and the milk. Simmer until the liquid has thickened to the consistency of heavy cream, 3 to 4 minutes. Mix in the rosemary, thyme, hot pepper sauce, and salt. Season the filling to taste with pepper. Transfer the filling to an oven-proof 6-cup baking dish.

6. Drain the cooked potatoes and place them in a large bowl. Mash them coarsely with a fork. Add the buttermilk and continue mashing until most of the lumps have been crushed. Blend in the mustard, then olive oil. Continue mashing until the potatoes are smooth and fluffy. Season them to taste with salt and pepper. Mix in the egg white.

7. Dollop the potatoes over the pot pie, covering it completely in an even layer. With the tines of a fork, make a decorative pattern in the potatoes.

8. Bake the pot pie until it is bubbling and the potatoes are golden, with lightly browned edges, 35 to 40 minutes. Let stand 10 minutes before serving.

OPTIONS: Use chicken in place of the turkey. Omit the mashed-potato topping and make this as a true pot pie by covering it with your favorite pie crust and baking until the crust is golden brown.

COOKING FOR TWO: You will enjoy this pot pie as leftovers in a day or two, which is good because, frankly, it is not worth your time to prepare this dish as a half recipe.

fillet of sole florentine

SERVES 4, 145 CALORIES, 2 GRAMS OF FAT PER SERVING.

The blend of herbs and vinegar in this dish is inspired by a recipe from the seventeenth century. It adds a piquant note to the combination of spinach and lean fish. Besides flavor, the herbs add useful phytochemicals, while the acid in the vinegar makes the iron in the spinach easier for your body to absorb.

    2 cups chopped fresh spinach
    ¼ cup dry bread crumbs
    1   tablespoon minced shallots
    ½ teaspoon mixed fresh rosemary, or ¼ teaspoon dry, crushed
    ½ teaspoon fresh thyme leaves, or ¼ teaspoon dry
    3 to 4 gratings fresh nutmeg, or pinch of ground
    ¼ teaspoon salt
    ¼ teaspoon freshly ground pepper
    1 pound fillet of sole, in 4 pieces
    ½ cup defatted chicken broth
    1 teaspoon cider vinegar
    1 teaspoon sugar
    Paprika, for garnish

1. Preheat the oven to 350°F.

2. In a large bowl, combine the spinach, bread crumbs, shallots, rosemary, thyme, nutmeg, salt, and pepper. Arrange the spinach mixture to cover the bottom of an 8-inch square or other shallow baking dish just large enough to hold the fish in one layer.

3. Arrange the pieces of fish over the spinach, overlapping them as little as possible.

4. In a small saucepan, combine the broth, vinegar, and sugar, and bring to a boil. Pour the hot liquid over the fish. Dust the fillets lightly with the paprika.

5. Bake until the fish is opaque white all the way through. Serve immediately.

halibut with garlic mashed potatoes

SERVES 4, 285 CALORIES, 11 GRAMS OF FAT PER SERVING.

The creamy texture and buttery flavor of yellow-fleshed potatoes such as Yukon Gold and Yellow Finn help you make fluffy, rich, yet lean mashed potatoes. Low-fat buttermilk is the secret for making them light. (The "butter" in its name is deceptive: True buttermilk is the lean liquid left after butter is churned. Now this tangy dairy product is usually made from low-fat or skim milk cultured with friendly bacteria.) Halibut is a mild-flavored fish. Its meaty, flaky white flesh contrasts perfectly with the velvety potatoes. Serve with Braised Fennel and Tomatoes (page. 285) or steamed string beans.

4 large yellow-fleshed potatoes, about ¾ pound, or 3 large russets, peeled and quartered
4 halibut steaks, each 4 ounces
2 tablespoons plus 1 teaspoon olive oil
3 cloves roasted garlic
⅓ cup low-fat buttermilk
Salt and freshly ground pepper to taste

1. Preheat the oven to 350°F.

2. Place the potatoes in a large pot and cover with cold water. Set over high heat until water boils. Reduce the heat to medium, cover, and cook until potatoes are easily pierced by a fork, 20 to 25 minutes.

3. After the potatoes have cooked for 15 minutes, coat the halibut with 1 teaspoon of the oil, using ¼ teaspoon per piece, or spray with cooking spray. Arrange the fish in a shallow baking pan large enough to hold them loosely. Bake the fish until it is opaque all the way through and just flakes when pierced with a fork, about 13 minutes. Set the fish aside, lightly covered with a piece of foil, while you mash the potatoes.

4. Drain the potatoes and turn them in a large bowl. With a fork, break up and start mashing the potatoes. Gradually add 1 tablespoon of the oil, the garlic, then the buttermilk, and salt to taste. Add the remaining oil and pepper to taste. Continue mashing until the potatoes are smooth and fluffy, 2 to 3 minutes.

5. To serve, flatten one cup of the potatoes on a dinner plate to make a bed. Place a piece of fish on the potatoes. Serve immediately.

OPTIONS: Serve leftover potatoes as a vegetable the next day, at room temperature or heated as a pancake in a skillet. Mix leftover potatoes into a broccoli soup.

COOKING FOR TWO: Use ½ pound of fish, cut into two pieces

sicilian spaghetti with swordfish

SERVES 4, 517 CALORIES, 10 GRAMS OF FAT PER SERVING.

Sicilians are blessed with great swordfish, intensely flavored sun-ripened tomatoes, superb olives, and the best capers in the world. Siracusans, in eastern Sicily, combine them all in this outstanding pasta dish. It is a memorable blending of energy foods and flavors, plus protective micronutrients including lycopene, beta- carotene, and more.

    1 tablespoon extra-virgin olive oil
    ½ cup finely chopped onion
    1 garlic clove, minced
    2 cups seeded and diced plum tomatoes (about 6)
    1 pound swordfish, cut in ¾-inch cubes
    1 teaspoon minced fresh rosemary, thyme, or oregano
    2 tablespoons chopped green Sicilian or Spanish olives
    1 tablespoon capers, drained and rinsed
    Pinch red pepper flakes
    Salt and freshly ground pepper to taste
    ¾ pound spaghetti
    1 tablespoon fresh lemon juice
    2 tablespoons chopped parsley

1. Bring to boil a large pot of water.

2. Heat the oil in a large, nonstick skillet, over medium-high heat. Sauté the onions and garlic until the onions soften, about 5 minutes.

3. Add the tomatoes and cook until they start to soften, 3 to 4 minutes, stirring occasionally.

4. Add the fish, herbs, olives, capers, red pepper flakes, salt, and freshly ground pepper to taste. Simmer gently until the fish is cooked through, about 8 minutes.

5. Meanwhile, cook the spaghetti according to package directions. Drain and place in a warm serving bowl.

6. Pour the sauce over the pasta. Sprinkle with the lemon juice and garnish with the parsley. Serve immediately.

salmon burgers

MAKES 4, 110 CALORIES, 4 GRAMS OF FAT PER SERVING.

The mashed potatoes used to bind these salmon cakes make them particularly light and delicate. The green beans add color and flavor; they also sneak in some fiber. Serve these burgers with boiled potatoes and steamed string beans dressed with vinaigrette.

½ pound fillet of salmon
¼ cup very thinly sliced green beans
2 tablespoons finely chopped chives
1 egg white, lightly beaten
2 tablespoons instant mashed potatoes
Pinch cayenne pepper
½ teaspoon salt
Freshly ground pepper

1. To separate the salmon from the skin, grasp a corner of the skin firmly with one hand. With the other hand, slip a knife horizontally between the flesh of the fish and the skin. (You may be able to ask your fish market to do this for you.) Discard the skin. Coarsely chop the salmon. Place it in a bowl.

2. Add the beans, chives, and egg white to the salmon. With a fork, stir to blend. The mixture will be quite wet. Mix in the mashed potatoes, salt, cayenne pepper, and a generous amount of freshly ground pepper. Form the mixture into 4 burgers, wetting your hands first with cold water. If not cooking them immediately, place the burgers on a plate, cover with foil, and refrigerate up to 24 hours.

3. Heat a nonstick skillet over medium-high heat. Add the salmon burgers, reduce the heat, and cook for 5 minutes. Turn and cook 5 minutes on the other side, until the fish is cooked and burgers are opaque all the way through.

shrimp with black bean salsa

SERVES 4, 290 CALORIES, 3 GRAMS OF FAT PER SERVING.

The large shrimp this dish recommends (smaller ones can be used and cooked for a slightly shorter time) are more expensive, but you'll find the elegant presentation makes them worth the cost. The citrus and seasonings in the salsa are so refreshing that no one will notice it is fat-free.

16 extra-large shrimp (10 to 12 count), about 1½ pounds
2 pink grapefruits
1 medium tomato, seeded and diced
1 medium (or pickling) cucumber, peeled and diced
½ cup diced red onion
¾ cup canned or cooked black beans
1 jalapeño or serrano chile pepper, seeded and minced
Juice of ½ orange
Juice of ½ lime
Salt and freshly ground pepper to taste
2 tablespoons chopped cilantro
1 tablespoon chopped mint

1. Cut the peel from the grapefruit. Holding the fruit over a medium bowl to catch the juices, release the sections from the membrane and collect them in the bowl. Cut the sections crosswise into 1-inch sections.

2. Add the diced tomato, cucumber, onion, beans, and chile pepper to the grapefruit and mix to blend. Pour in the orange and lime juice. Season to taste with salt and freshly ground pepper. Set aside.

3. Boil a large pot of water. Add the shrimp. When the water returns to a boil, cook the shrimp until they are pink, curled, and opaque all the way through, 6 to 8 minutes. Drain immediately. As soon as the shrimp are cool enough to handle, peel and devein them.

4. Place the shrimp on a cutting board and slit them horizontally along the back, cutting almost all the way through, but not completely, from the tip to the tail.

5. Arrange 4 shrimp in a pinwheel, tails inside, on each of 4 dinner plates. Spoon a tablespoon of the salsa into the slit in each shrimp. Mound the remaining salsa in the center of the plate, covering the tails of the shrimp. Sprinkle a quarter of the cilantro and mint over each plate and serve immediately.

black bean stew with pineapple

SERVES 4, 214 CALORIES, 3 GRAMS OF FAT PER SERVING.

Call this a meatless chili with a Caribbean glow. Yellow-skinned ripe plantain and fresh pineapple add fiber along with the unexpected appeal of sweet and sour notes to this easy-to-assemble dish. It is a good choice to make on Sunday and enjoy for several days.

    2 teaspoons canola oil
    ½ cup white or yellow onion, finely chopped
    1 medium green bell pepper, seeded and chopped
    2 garlic cloves, minced
    1 jalapeño or serrano chile pepper, seeded and minced (optional)
    2 plum tomatoes, seeded and chopped
    ½ cup thinly sliced fresh pineapple (see note on page 259)
    ½ ripe plantain, cut in ½-inch slices
    15-ounce can black beans, drained and rinsed
    1 teaspoon ground cumin
    ⅛ teaspoon ground allspice
    ½ cup vegetable broth or water
    Salt and freshly ground pepper to taste
    Chopped cilantro, for garnish

1. In a small Dutch oven, heat the oil over medium-high heat. Sauté the onions, bell peppers, and garlic until the onions are translucent, 4 to 5 minutes. Add the jalapeño, tomatoes, pineapples, plantains, and beans. Stir in the cumin and allspice and cook 1 to 2 minutes. Add the broth or water and

simmer the stew 15 minutes, until the flavors have blended and the plantains are tender. Season with salt and pepper, if needed. Serve over cooked brown or white rice.

NOTE: For a small amount of fresh pineapple, check the salad bar at your supermarket. Also check the produce department, where you may find a package of sliced, fresh pineapple. If neither is available and you do not want to buy a whole pineapple, get a can of pineapple rings and cut a couple of them into thin slices.

OPTIONS: Use frozen, canned, or fresh corn kernels in place of the pineapple and plantains. Use banana to replace the plantain. Mix in cooked, cubed turkey or chicken.

COOKING FOR TWO: Bring leftovers to room temperature and mix with cooked rice to serve as a main dish salad.

creole stuffed peppers

SERVES 4, 281 CALORIES, 7 GRAMS OF FAT PER SERVING.

The rice filling in stuffed peppers can be heavy and wet. Here, brown basmati rice stays fluffy and light. The combination of beans, corn, feta cheese, and onions added to the vitamin C–rich peppers and whole-grain rice make this dish a hefty source of both nutrients and energy. This meatless main course also provides satisfyingly intense flavor.

- 4 medium green peppers
- 2 cups cooked brown basmati-type rice
- 1 cup canned pinto beans
- ¾ cup finely chopped onion
- ¾ cup frozen, canned, or fresh corn kernels
- ½ cup (2 ounces) crumbled feta cheese
- 1½ teaspoons dried basil
- Salt and freshly ground pepper to taste
- 2 teaspoons extra-virgin olive oil
- 1 tablespoon fresh lemon juice

1. Preheat the oven to 375°F. Spray an 8-inch square baking dish with cooking spray.

2. Cut the tops off the peppers and seed them. Reserve the tops. If necessary, to help the peppers stand firmly, trim a bit off the bottom, taking care not to cut through to the inside. Set aside.

3. In a large bowl, combine the rice, beans, onion, corn, feta, and basil. Season to taste with salt and freshly ground pepper.

4. Spoon the filling into the peppers, packing it lightly and mounding it nicely over the top. Place the peppers in the baking dish and cover with the reserved tops. Place the baking dish in the center of the oven and add water to a depth of 1½ inches.

5. Bake until the peppers are soft when pierced with a knife, about one hour. Remove the pepper tops and discard. In a small bowl, combine the olive oil and lemon juice. Spoon this mixture over the hot peppers. Let sit 20 minutes and serve.

OPTIONS: Use 3 ounces (½ can) tuna in place of the feta cheese. If peppers disagree with you, make the filling only, adding ¼ cup chicken or vegetable broth. Bake, covered with foil, for 30 minutes and serve.

COOKING FOR TWO: This recipe can be halved.

moroccan stuffed onions

SERVES 4, 197 CALORIES, 3 GRAMS OF FAT PER SERVING.

Onions are a great source of allicin, so dishes featuring them are good cancer fighters. Their flavor is also most appealing, especially when roasting brings out their natural sweetness. Stuffed onions are popular throughout the Mediterranean. Here, a Moroccan blend of spices along with chickpeas and light-textured brown basmati rice turns these onions into a lovely main dish.

    4 medium onions
1½ cups cooked brown basmati or plain rice

½ cup cooked chickpeas
3 tablespoons dried currants
2 tablespoons chopped parsley
1 tablespoon fresh lemon juice
½ tablespoon fresh ground cumin
¼ teaspoon paprika
¼ teaspoon ground cinnamon
1 cup chicken broth
1 teaspoon extra-virgin olive oil
Salt and freshly ground pepper to taste
1 tablespoon white wine vinegar

1. Peel the onions. Cut off the tops at the point where the sides curve in towards the top. Cook the onions in a large pot of boiling water for 2 minutes. With a slotted spoon, remove the onions from the pot.

2. When the onions are cool enough to handle, use a melon baller to scoop out the flesh, leaving a shell 2 layers thick.

3. Preheat oven to 375°F.

4. In a medium bowl, combine the rice, chickpeas, currants, parsley, lemon juice, cumin, paprika, cinnamon, and salt and pepper. Pack the mixture into the onions.

5. Place the onions in an 8-inch square baking dish. Pour in the chicken broth. Drizzle the onions with the olive oil. Bake at 375°F until the onions are tender when pierced with a knife, about 30 minutes. Set the onions on a serving plate. Pour the cooking liquid into a small pot.

6. Add the vinegar and boil the liquid until it is reduced to ¼ cup. Pour 1 tablespoon of this liquid over each onion, and serve.

lentil and mushroom stew

SERVES 6, 281 CALORIES, 3 GRAMS OF FAT PER SERVING.

Mushrooms add more than meaty flavor to dishes; they are also a rich source of cancer-preventing terpines. Here, keeping the mushrooms firm also enhances the texture of this appealing Mediterranean meatless dish. Serve it with roasted red-skinned new potatoes and a green salad lightly drizzled with olive oil.

2 cups green lentils
½ cup dried porcini mushrooms
2 teaspoons olive oil
½ cup chopped onion
½ cup chopped leek
2 cups quartered white mushrooms
2 cloves roasted garlic
¾ cup Rich Vegetable Stock (page 240)
2 teaspoons red wine vinegar
1 teaspoon minced fresh rosemary, or ½ teaspoon dried
1 bay leaf
Salt and freshly ground pepper to taste

1. In a deep saucepan, bring 3½ cups water to a boil. Add the lentils and cook until tender, about 25 minutes.

2. Soak the porcini mushrooms in a small bowl in warm water to cover until they are soft, 20 to 30 minutes.

3. In a small Dutch oven, heat the oil over medium-high heat. Sauté the onions and leeks until the onions are translucent, about five minutes. Add the white mushrooms and cook until they give off their liquid. Add the vegetable stock then the drained porcini mushrooms, garlic, lentils, rosemary, and bay leaf. Season to taste with salt and pepper.

4. Bring the stew to a boil, reduce the heat, and simmer gently until the white mushrooms are cooked through. If possible, let sit 1 to 2 hours and reheat before serving.

texas quick-step chili for two

SERVES 2, 437 CALORIES, 7 GRAMS OF FAT PER SERVING.

Chili makes a great meatless meal. Full of fire and fiber, it is filling and fulfilling to eat. Most chili recipes make enough to feed an army, albeit a small one. When you don't want to eat it for a week, or pack portions away in the freezer, here is the answer. Cooking the feisty, flavorful base first, then adding cooked beans near the end, reverses the typical order in chili-making. It also speeds the process considerably. Don't discard your favorite chili recipe, but when dinner needs to be on the table, and it's a table for two, this distinctive method satisfies for taste, time, and quality.

    2 teaspoons canola oil
    ½ cup chopped onion
    ½ cup chopped green bell pepper
    1 garlic clove, chopped
    1 small jalapeno pepper, seeded and minced
    1 teaspoon ground cumin
    14½-ounce can diced tomatoes, with their liquid, or 2 cups canned
        tomatoes, broken up
    1 teaspoon diced oregano
    1 tablespoon chopped cilantro
    15-ounce can pinto beans, rinsed and drained, or 2 cups cooked beans
    1 corn tortilla, torn into 1-inch pieces
    Freshly ground pepper

1. In a small Dutch oven, heat the oil over medium-high heat. Saute the onions, green pepper, and garlic until the onions are soft, 6 to 7 minutes. Mix in the jalapeño and cumin and cook, stirring constantly, until the cumin is aromatic, about 30 seconds.

2. Add the tomatoes, oregano, and cilantro, reduce the heat to medium, and simmer for 10 minutes, until the mixture thickens slightly.

3. Add the beans, tortilla, and freshly ground pepper to taste. Simmer gently in the sauce for 10 minutes. Let the chili sit 10 to 20 minutes before serving, or cook and refrigerate, then reheat and serve.

lasagna con verdura

SERVES 8, 399 CALORIES, 15 GRAMS OF FAT PER SERVING.

This is the lightest lasagna you can imagine. Layers of vegetables and cheese bathed in a lean bechamel sauce give it Mediterannean elegance. Use precooked lasagna noodles to cut time and work. This is a delightful way to make sure everyone eats their veggies at a potluck party or at home.

1   small eggplant, cut lengthwise into ¼-inch slices
2   cups 2-percent milk
3   tablespoons flour
3   cups shredded part-skim-milk mozzarella cheese
¾   cup finely chopped onion
¾   cup chopped zucchini
1¼ cups chopped mushrooms
½   cup defatted chicken broth
10-ounce package frozen chopped spinach, defrosted and squeezed dry
15 ounces reduced-fat ricotta cheese
¼   cup low-fat buttermilk
1½ cups fat-free pasta sauce
9   precooked lasagna noodles
1   tablespoon grated Parmesan cheese
2   teaspoons dry bread crumbs
Salt and freshly ground pepper to taste

1. Preheat oven to 375°F.

2. Spray a baking sheet liberally with cooking spray. Arrange the eggplant on the pan and coat with cooking spray. Bake until the eggplant is soft, 12 to 15 minutes. Let cool on the baking sheet. (This step can be done up to one day ahead.) Reduce oven to 350°F.

3. For the white sauce: In a saucepan, heat 1½ cups of the milk until it steams. In a small bowl whisk the remaining milk into the flour.

4. Whisk the flour mixture into the hot milk. Cook until the sauce thickens and just comes to a boil. Remove from the heat and stir in 2 cups of the mozzarella. Season to taste with salt and pepper. Set aside.

5. Spray a medium, nonstick skillet with cooking spray and place the pan over medium-high heat. Add the onions, zucchini, and mushrooms, and sauté until the onions soften, about 6 minutes, stirring often. Add the chicken broth and simmer, uncovered, over medium heat, until the vegetables are tender-crisp, about 8 minutes. Stir in the spinach, season to taste with salt and pepper. Set aside.

6. In a bowl, combine the ricotta cheese with the remaining cup of mozzarella, and add the buttermilk. Season to taste with salt and freshly ground pepper. Set aside.

7. To assemble the lasagna: Spread 1 cup of the pasta sauce to cover the bottom of a 9- inch x 13-inch baking dish. Cover with 3 pieces of the lasagna noodles, taking care they do not overlap. Cover with the eggplant and remaining ½ cup pasta sauce. Top with 3 more of the noodles. Spread ½ cup of the white sauce over the pasta. Spread the vegetable mixture over this and top with another ½ cup white sauce. Cover with another layer of pasta. Spread the prepared cheese mixture over the pasta. Cover with the remaining white sauce.

8. In a small bowl, combine the Parmesan cheese with the bread crumbs. Sprinkle over the lasagna. Cover the lasagna with foil.

9. Bake the lasagna covered for 20 minutes. Uncover and bake 10 minutes. Remove from oven and let stand 10 minutes.

light meals and salads

spinach and pink grapefruit salad

SERVES 4, 50 CALORIES, 2 GRAMS OF FAT PER SERVING.

Deep emerald spinach and blushing pink grapefruit are an ideal combination because the vitamin C in the fruit makes the iron in the greens more available to your body. Another good reason to enjoy this salad is because the combination of citrus fruit and greens, sprinkled with fresh basil, is so refreshing. Prepare all the elements of this salad up to a day ahead, then assemble them just before serving.

    6 cups loosely packed tender spinach leaves, stemmed
    8 large (about ⅓ cup) fresh basil leaves, cut crosswise in ¼-inch
         strips 1 tablespoon minced shallot
    1 medium pink grapefruit
    1 teaspoon olive oil
    Salt and freshly ground pepper to taste

1. In a salad bowl, toss the spinach with the basil and shallots.

2. Peel and section the grapefruit: Slice off the top and bottom of the grapefruit. Cut the peel and white part away by slicing it off in vertical strips, turning the grapefruit as you cut. Hold the peeled grapefruit over a bowl to catch the juices. Free each segment by slipping a small knife vertically along the membrane on each side.

3. Arrange 8 of the grapefruit sections over the spinach. Reserve the rest of the fruit for another use.

4. For the dressing, in a small bowl combine 2 tablespoons of juice from the grapefruit with the olive oil. Season to taste with salt and pepper.

5. Toss the salad with the dressing and serve immediately.

OPTIONS: Crumble a tablespoon of feta cheese over each serving of salad, warm the salad gently in a skillet until the spinach is just wilted and use it as a vegetable, accompanying baked sole or flounder.

COOKING FOR TWO: Use 3 cups of spinach and 4 grapefruit sections. Serve extra dressing as a vinaigrette over a crisp green salad.

quinoa tabbouleh

SERVES 4, 150 CALORIES, 5 GRAMS OF FAT PER SERVING.

Typically, tabbouleh is made from bulgur wheat, but quinoa or millet can be used to make lighter versions. Quinoa, a South American grain, is also higher in protein than wheat. Rinse it well before cooking to be sure all of the bitter-tasting coating, naturally found on this grain, is gone.

    2 cups cooked quinoa
    ½ cup green bell pepper, cut in ½-inch dice
    ½ cup chopped tomato, seeded and cut in ½-inch dice
    ⅓ cup chopped radish, cut in ½-inch dice
    2 scallions (¼ cup) green and white part, chopped
    2 tablespoons chopped mint
    2 tablespoons chopped Italian parsley
    Juice of ½ lime
    1 tablespoon extra virgin olive oil
    Salt and freshly ground pepper to taste

1. In a large bowl, combine the quinoa with the pepper, tomato, radishes, scallion, mint, and parsley. Add the lime juice and oil and toss to combine. Season to taste with salt and freshly ground pepper.

OPTIONS: You can add or subtract easily with this recipe. For example, use twice the amount of parsley and omit the mint, or use ¼ cup of red onion in place of the scallion.

COOKING FOR TWO: Halve the quantities given, or keep any leftovers. They will be good for about 2 days.

red bean and rice salad

SERVES 4, 230 CALORIES, 1 GRAM OF FAT PER SERVING.

Unpolished versions of rices like basmati and Texmati are light and delicately flavored. Combined with canned kidney beans, this whole-grain rice makes an appealing salad. Mango here adds carotenoids along with sunny tropical flavor.

> 2 cups cooked brown rice, such as basmati or Texmati
> 15-ounce can red kidney beans, drained and rinsed
> ¾ cup finely chopped green bell pepper
> ½ cup fresh mango, cut in ½-inch cubes
> ½ cup finely chopped red onion
> ½ cup salsa
> Salt and freshly ground pepper to taste
> 2 tablespoons chopped cilantro

1. In a large bowl, use a fork to combine the rice, beans, pepper, mango, and onion. Drain the salsa well and mix it into the salad. Season to taste with salt and freshly ground pepper.

2. Just before serving, sprinkle with the cilantro. This salad keeps 2 to 3 days, but the rice gets hard when refrigerated.

OPTIONS: Include a minced jalapeño or serrano pepper, if you like heat. Use diced, seeded fresh tomato in place of the mango, with lime juice in place of the salsa.

COOKING FOR TWO: Use half the amount of each ingredients.

mexican chicken salad

SERVES 4, 180 CALORIES, 2 GRAMS OF FAT PER SERVING.

- 1 pound jicama
- 2 cups (about 8 ounces) diced cooked chicken breast
- 1 navel orange
- ½ cup thin cucumber slices, halved into crescents
- ¼ cup thinly sliced red onion, in crescents
- 4 teaspoons olive oil
- ¼ cup freshly squeezed orange juice
- 2 tablespoons freshly squeezed lime juice
- 1 teaspoon salt
- 4 cups romaine lettuce, torn in 2-inch pieces
- ¼ teaspoon (round) ancho chili powder, or 3 to 4 dashes hot pepper sauce
- 2 tablespoons coarsely chopped cilantro

1. Peel the jicama. Cut it crosswise into ½-inch rounds. Stacking 2 to 3 rounds at a time, cut them crosswise into strips ½-inch wide. Cut the longest strips into 2-inch pieces. Place the cut-up jicama in a large, nonreactive glass, plastic, or stainless steel bowl. Add the chicken.

2. Peel and thinly slice the orange. Cut the slices into quarters. Add them to the bowl. Add the cucumber and onion.

3. In a small bowl, whisk together the oil, orange and lime juices, and salt. Mix until blended. If using hot sauce, add it at this point. Pour the dressing over the chicken salad and toss to blend.

4. Arrange 1 cup of the lettuce on each of four salad plates. Heap a quarter of the chicken salad on each plate. Sprinkle with the chili powder and the cilantro. Serve immediately. This salad is best when freshly made, but it can keep about an hour; after that the citrus flavors fade.

OPTIONS: In place of the sliced orange, use 1 cup seeded and diced tomato. If jicama is not available, use 1 cup of thinly sliced white daikon or regular red radishes.

COOKING FOR TWO: Make half the recipe, saving the unused part of the jicama to slice and serve as crudités.

tuna waldorf salad

SERVES 4, 135 CALORIES, 5 GRAMS OF FAT PER SERVING.

Waldorf salad may seem quaintly old-fashioned, but it is full of up-to-date good nutrition, with the apples, grapes, and walnuts adding valuable flavonoids and ellagic acid. Combining yogurt with mayonnaise, both low-fat versions of course, lightens the dressing nicely.

  6½-ounce can water-packed tuna, drained
  1 rib celery, cut in ½-inch dice
  ½ Granny Smith apple, peeled, cored, and cut in ½-inch dice
  ½ cup halved seedless red grapes
  2 tablespoons chopped walnuts
  2 tablespoons low-fat mayonnaise
  2 tablespoons fat-free plain yogurt
  1 tablespoon fresh lemon juice
  Salt and freshly ground pepper to taste

1. In a bowl, flake the tuna. Add the celery, apple, grapes, and walnuts and mix to combine.

2. Mix in the mayonnaise, yogurt and lemon juice until the salad is well blended. Season to taste with salt and pepper. This salad keeps up to 24 hours, tightly covered, in the refrigerator.

OPTIONS: Use raisins in place of the walnuts. Add 1 teaspoon curry powder along with the dressing.

COOKING FOR TWO: You can use a small can of tuna and halve the amounts of the other ingredients, but this salad keeps well, so why not make the entire recipe?

creamy tonnato dressing

MAKES ABOUT 1 CUP, SERVES ABOUT 6, 47 CALORIES, LESS THAN 1 GRAM OF FAT PER SERVING.

In Italy, canned tuna is pureed to make a mayonnaise-based sauce that is the key to Vitello Tonnato, a lovely cold dish. Since the tuna provides protein, why not turn this sauce into a salad dressing that, in turn, transforms a crisp green salad into a complete, light main dish? Enjoy it over a combination of romaine and green leaf lettuces, sliced cucumber, and red bell pepper.

6¼-ounce can chunk light tuna in water
4 anchovy fillets, rinsed and dried
1 garlic clove
1 tablespoon capers, rinsed and dried
2 tablespoons fat-free mayonnaise
Pinch cayenne pepper
6 tablespoons defatted low-sodium chicken broth
1 tablespoon red wine vinegar
Freshly ground pepper to taste

1. In a food processor, process the tuna with the anchovies, garlic, and capers until they are very finely chopped. Add the mayonnaise and cayenne and process until very well blended.

2. Pour in the chicken broth and vinegar. Process until the dressing has the texture of stirred yogurt. Season to taste with the pepper. This dressing keeps, refrigerated in a tightly closed container, for 2 to 3 days.

turkey and avocado wrap

MAKES 1, 256 CALORIES, 8 GRAMS OF FAT.

Here is an updated version of a favorite sandwich. The layers of filling are arranged so that this wrap keeps well up to 24 hours. This means you can make it the night before to put in a lunch bag or pack on a picnic. Creamy avocado is a delicious source of beneficial monounsaturated fat.

- 1 9-inch whole-wheat tortilla
- 1 tablespoon fat-free mayonnaise
- 2 ounces thinly sliced turkey breast
- 4 thin tomato slices
- 1 to 2 teaspoons minced jalapeño
- 2 tablespoons shredded low-fat cheddar cheese
- 1 teaspoon minced cilantro
- 2 ½-inch wedges avocado

1. Lay the tortilla on a cutting board and spread the two-thirds nearest you with mayonnaise.

2. Cover the same area with sliced turkey. Lay the tomato over the turkey. Sprinkle with the jalapeño, cheese, and cilantro. Place the avocado wedges across the bottom of the tortilla, two inches away from the edge.

3. Fold the bottom of the tortilla up over the avocado. Fold the two sides in. Pull at the bottom. To keep the filling from pushing forward, keep pulling the rolled part toward you. This also helps make a firm roll.

OPTIONS: Replace the sliced tomato with a very well-drained, prepared chunky salsa.

chicken fajitas

SERVES 4, 179 CALORIES, 4 GRAMS OF FAT PER SERVING.

Instead of grilled chicken, here it is sautéed and nestled in a tortilla with browned onions and crisp, tender green peppers spiked with jalapeños. The cumin, which gives these fajitas bold flavor, also contains curcumin, which may help lower the risk for certain cancers. Serve with Red-Bean and Rice Salad (page 268) or fiber-rich refried beans.

Juice of ½ lime
1 whole boneless, skinless chicken breast
1 teaspoon ground cumin
2 teaspoons canola oil
½ large white onion, thinly sliced
1 medium green bell pepper, seeded, cut in ½-inch strips
1 to 2 jalapeño peppers, seeded, cut lengthwise in thin strips
4 9-inch wheat tortillas
¼ cup well-drained salsa
2 tablespoons chopped cilantro

1. Pour the lime juice into a plastic container just large enough to hold the chicken breast. Sprinkle the cumin over the chicken, being sure to season it on both sides. Place the seasoned breast in the container and marinate in the refrigerator, 2 to 24 hours.

2. Add one teaspoon of the oil to a medium, nonstick skillet set over medium-high heat. Add the onion, green and jalapeño peppers, stirring to coat them with the oil. Sauté until the onions are lightly browned, about 15 minutes. The peppers will still be slightly crisp. Set aside. Do not clean the pan.

3. Cut the marinated chicken lengthwise into 10 to 12 strips, the thinner the better. In the pan used to sauté the vegetables, heat the remaining oil. Add the chicken and cook until no pink shows in the center of the thickest piece, about 4 minutes on each side. The meat may brown slightly.

4. Place 2 to 3 chicken slices in the center of a tortilla. Add one tablespoon of the drained salsa and a quarter of the sautéed vegetables. Sprinkle generously with the cilantro. Roll this filling in the tortilla and serve immediately.

OPTIONS: Add grated fat-free cheddar and avocado in place of the onions and peppers.

COOKING FOR TWO: Marinate half a chicken breast. Reduce the amounts of the other ingredients accordingly.

roasted vegetable wrap

SERVES 4, 165 CALORIES, 6 GRAMS OF FAT PER SERVING.

This wrap puts an aromatic assortment of roasted vegetables right in your hands, making it easy to take generous servings of vegetables along on a picnic, or to pack them in a lunch bag. The goat cheese adds flavor and calcium. Be as generous as you like with the roasted garlic, it can only do you good.

1 small eggplant
3 teaspoons extra-virgin olive oil
½ small bulb fennel, cut vertically in very thin slices
2 large mushrooms, thinly sliced
1 small zucchini, thinly sliced
1 small red pepper, seeded and cut in ¼-inch strips
8 thin slices red onion
8 to 12 whole cloves garlic, peeled
2 teaspoons minced fresh rosemary, or ½ teaspoon dried and crushed
15-inch piece soft cracker bread, or two 9-inch wheat tortillas
2 tablespoons soft, fresh goat cheese
Salt and freshly ground pepper to taste

1. Preheat oven to 375°F. Spray two baking sheets with cooking spray.

2. Cut 4 ¼-inch-thick slices vertically from the eggplant. Set aside the remaining eggplant for another use. Lay the slices, in one layer, on one of the prepared baking sheets. Pour ½ teaspoon of the olive oil on your palm, rub it over the slices, turning so both sides are lightly coated. Do the same with the fennel. Arrange both vegetables on one baking sheet. Roast until the eggplant is tender, 12 to 15 minutes.

3. Meanwhile, in a bowl, toss the mushrooms and zucchini with the second teaspoon of oil. Arrange in one layer on the second baking sheet. Roast until tender, about 10 minutes. Set aside.

4. Toss the red pepper, onion, and garlic with the remaining oil, salt and pepper, and the rosemary. Reusing the baking sheet from the eggplant, spread the vegetables in one layer and roast until softened, about 15 minutes. Set aside.

5. To assemble one wrap, spread a quarter of the cheese to thinly cover one side of the bread completely. Arrange a quarter of the vegetables to cover two-thirds of the bread, keeping the cheese-only part at the top, starting with the eggplant. Cover this with a layer of the fennel, followed by one of the red pepper mixture. Top with a layer of the mushrooms and zucchini.

6. Roll up the filled bread, jelly-roll fashion, starting at the bottom. To keep the filling from pushing forward, keep pulling the rolled part toward you. This also helps to make a firm roll. Wrap the roll in plastic wrap and refrigerate from 4 to 48 hours. To serve, cut into 2-inch slices.

OPTIONS: Use whole-wheat pita breads in place of the cracker bread or tortillas to make more transportable sandwiches.

COOKING FOR TWO: **Make all the vegetables.** Use the extra as a side dish over the next day or two.

stuffed portobello mushrooms

SERVES 4, 182 CALORIES, 5 GRAMS OF FAT PER SERVING.

These grain-stuffed mushrooms, a meatless equivalent of meat and potatoes, are as naturally classy a combination as Ginger Rodgers and Fred Astaire. Kasha, a grain that cooks quickly, is an invaluable source of flavenoids. The dill and mushrooms add terpenes. Buttermilk tops off all the flavors in the filling with just the right note.

1¼ cups defatted chicken broth
½ cup whole toasted buckwheat (kasha)
1 tablespoon olive oil
5 large portobello mushrooms, steamed
1 cup finely chopped onion
1 cup peeled potato, cut in ½-inch cubes
¼ cup low-fat buttermilk
Salt and freshly ground pepper to taste
Chopped dill, for garnish (optional)

1. Cook the buckwheat: In a medium saucepan, combine the chicken broth with 1 cup water and bring to a boil. Stir in the kasha and 1 teaspoon of oil. Cover, and cook over medium heat for 12 minutes, until the kasha is done. Remove from the heat and let sit, covered, 5 minutes. Uncover and fluff with fork. Set aside.

2. Cook the mushrooms: Spray a large, nonstick skillet liberally with cooking spray and place the pan over medium-high heat. Add 4 of the mushrooms, top-side down, and cook until lightly browned, 5 to 7 minutes. Turn and cook until the mushrooms are tender but not soft. Set them on a plate, gill-side down, to drain. Wipe out the pan.

3. Make the filling: Finely chop the remaining mushroom. Add the remaining oil to the pan. Over medium-high heat, sauté the onion, potatoes, and chopped mushroom until the potatoes are tender and the liquid from the mushroom has evaporated, 15 to 18 minutes. Mix in the buttermilk and stir until the filling clumps when pressed with a spoon. Remove from the heat and season to taste with salt and freshly ground pepper.

4. Arrange the mushrooms, gills up, on a serving plate. Pack the filling into the

mushrooms, mounding it nicely. Serve immediately, sprinkled with the dill.

NOTE: This recipe can be made up to 8 hours ahead, then reheated in a microwave oven.

OPTIONS: Add a minced garlic clove, minced shallot, or teaspoon of chopped fresh rosemary to the filling, if you wish, when sautéing the onions. Serve any leftover filling the next day as a side dish.

COOKING FOR TWO: Use half the cooked buckwheat, and cut the amount of the other ingredients by half. Heat the unused buckwheat with milk and maple syrup for breakfast.

polenta stew

SERVES 4, 246 CALORIES, 11 GRAMS OF FAT PER SERVING.

Polenta is often served with a topping, but here cubes of polenta are simmered in a chunky, flavorful tomato sauce. This stew, a whole-grain alternative to a bowl of pasta, is such a satisfying dish that you may want to start from scratch. This is simple with oven-baked polenta.

```
2  tablespoons extra-virgin olive oil
1  cup finely chopped onion
1  chopped clove garlic
28-ounce can plum tomatoes, drained
1  teaspoon dried oregano
2  sun-dried tomato halves, finely chopped
1  tablespoon salt and freshly ground pepper to taste
1  recipe Oven-Baked Polenta (page 278), at room temperature
2  tablespoons grated Parmesan cheese
```

1. In a large, deep saucepan or small Dutch oven, heat the oil over medium-high heat. Sauté the onion and garlic until softened, 5 minutes.

2. Add the plum tomatoes, oregano, and sun-dried tomatoes. Season to taste with salt and pepper. Simmer until the tomatoes are soft but not mushy, about 15 minutes.

3. Meanwhile, cut the polenta into 1-inch cubes. Add it to the sauce, stirring gently so the polenta holds its shape. Simmer just until the polenta is heated through. Serve sprinkled with the grated cheese.

OPTIONS: Brown the meat from one large link of freshly made Italian sausage and sauté it in the sauce along with the tomatoes. Mix ½ cup reduced-fat mozzarella cheese, cut in ½-inch cubes, into the hot stew just before serving.

COOKING FOR TWO: Make the entire sauce recipe, but remove half and set aside for another use. Add half a recipe of Oven-Baked Polenta.

oven-baked polenta

SERVES 6, 71 CALORIES, 2 GRAMS OF FAT PER SERVING.

Normally, you have to stand and stir polenta as it cools, but chefs like Gary Danko from San Francisco have found this hands-off way to make it in the oven. It's so effortless that you can enjoy this Italianate cornmeal mush often. If you use imported polenta, avoid the instant kind. Stone-ground yellow cornmeal makes a smoother polenta and has the additional advantage of including the germ of the corn. Serve topped with Garlic Greens (page 286), tomato sauce, or a sprinkling of grated Parmesan cheese.

    2 teaspoons olive oil
    ¾ cup polenta or yellow stone-ground cornmeal
    3 cups boiling water
    ¼ cup finely chopped onion
    ½ teaspoon salt

1. Preheat oven to 350°F.

2. In a medium cast-iron or other heavy, oven-proof pot, heat the oil over medium-high heat. With a wooden spoon, mix in the polenta, stirring until it is coated with oil and hot to the touch, about 5 minutes. Reduce the heat, if necessary, to avoid browning. Turn off the heat.

3. Stand back and carefully whisk the boiling water into the polenta mixture. The mixture will splutter and spatter. Keep whisking until the polenta is smooth. Mix in the onions and salt.

4. Place the polenta in the oven, uncovered. Bake 45 minutes, until it is thick and slightly grainy but tender to the bite.

5. Meanwhile, coat a 9-inch square baking dish with oil or cooking spray. Pour the hot polenta into the prepared dish, scraping as much of it as you can from the pot. Smooth the polenta with a moistened rubber spatula to make an even layer. Set it aside to cool. (See Note below.)

6. Cover the cooled polenta and refrigerate until ready to use. It keeps 2 to 3 days in the refrigerator. To serve, cut into squares, wrap in foil and heat in 350%F oven until hot. Or sauté in a nonstick skillet, using 1 to 2 teaspoons olive oil. Cook until the polenta is crisp on the outside and heated through.

NOTE: A certain amount of cooked polenta will always stick to the pot. Rather than using elbow grease, use this simple trick to clean the pot. As soon as you have poured out the polenta, place the hot pot in the sink, fill it with cold water and let it soak. When the pot has cooled, you will find the coating of polenta stuck to it has released. Without scrubbing, you can empty it out with the cold soaking water.

COOKING FOR TWO: Extra polenta can be reheated in the oven or crisped in a skillet, using a bit of olive oil or cooking spray.

salmon-stuffed baked potato

MAKES 4, 194 CALORIES, 6 GRAMS OF FAT PER SERVING.

This is an easy way to add an interesting new taste to the old standby baked potato. The use of salmon in this easy recipe also adds the cancer protection of omega-3 fatty acids to your menu.

2 large (¾ pound) russet potatoes
7-½-ounce can red salmon
1 tablespoon pesto
Freshly ground pepper to taste
2 tablespoons chopped Italian parsley

1. Preheat the oven to 400°F.

2. Bake the potatoes until soft when squeezed, about 45 minutes.

3. While the potatoes bake, place the salmon in a small bowl. Remove all the skin and the large bones. With a fork, mash the salmon and blend in the pesto. Season generously with the pepper. Mix in the parsley.

4. When the potatoes are done, cut them in half lengthwise. Place each half in a cereal-size bowl. With a fork, mash and fluff the flesh of the potato. Add a quarter of the salmon to each bowl, partially blending it with the fluffed potato, and serve.

broccoli-stuffed baked potato

SERVES 2, 276 CALORIES, 2 GRAMS OF FAT PER SERVING.

The overall health benefits of broccoli have been well documented, especially in terms of cancer protection. This easy recipe combines the values of this cruciferous vegetable with the solid nutrition and good taste of potatoes for a sidedish or meatless main dish everyone will enjoy.

    2 large (¾ pound) russet potatoes
    1 large stalk fresh broccoli, or 10-ounce package frozen chopped
    ½ bouillon cube
    ½ cup (2 ounces) reduced-fat Swiss cheese, finely chopped
    ½ teaspoon dried oregano
    Freshly ground pepper to taste

1. Preheat the oven to 400°F.

2. Bake the potatoes until soft when squeezed.

3. If using fresh broccoli, separate the buds from the stalk, cutting them off as closely as possible to make small clusters. Place florets in a bowl. Finely chop the small stems just below the florets and set aside. With a small, sharp knife, cut off the tough bottom of the thick broccoli stem. Starting at the top and cutting the length of the stem, cut away the tough outer part of the stalk. Much of it will be pared away, leaving the heart, a stick about 4 to 5 inches long by about 1 inch. Chop this up.

4. Place all the chopped stems in a medium saucepan. Add ½ cup water and the bouillon. Over medium-high heat, cook the broccoli, tightly covered, for 5 minutes. Add the florets and cook 5 minutes longer, until all the broccoli is soft. If using frozen chopped broccoli, cook according to package directions until it is very soft.

5. When the potatoes are done, cut them in half lengthwise. Place each in a cereal-size bowl. With a fork, mash and fluff the flesh of the potato. Spoon half the broccoli over each potato. Add half the cheese to each, and sprinkle with half the oregano. With the fork, mash the broccoli and cheese with the potato flesh until the cheese is softened. Season to taste with pepper, and serve.

whole wheat bread with fresh herbs

MAKES 1 LOAF, ABOUT 10 SLICES, 117 CALORIES, 3 GRAMS OF FAT PER SLICE.

Most quick breads are sweet, like zucchini bread. Here, a generous helping of fresh herbs goes into an unusual, savory loaf. Slice this chewy, wonderfully aromatic bread and top it with a slab of ripe red tomato, or cover it with a slice of mozarella cheese and grill. Toasted, it is good spread with Radish and Cucumber Raita (page 295).

½ cup white bread flour
1 cup whole wheat flour
½ cup rolled oats (not quick-cooking or instant)
½ teaspoon baking soda
½ teaspoon salt
½ teaspoon freshly ground black pepper
¼ cup chopped parsley
¼ cup chopped scallion, green part only
2 tablespoons chopped fresh basil
2 eggs, lightly beaten
1 cup low-fat buttermilk
1 tablespoon extra-virgin olive oil

1. Preheat the oven to 375°F. Spray a 9-inch x 5-inch x 2-½-inch loaf pan with cooking spray.

2. In a large bowl, combine the two flours, oats, baking soda, and salt and pepper. Mix in the parsley, scallions, and basil.

3. In a small bowl, lightly beat the eggs. Mix in the buttermilk and oil until well combined.

4. Add the wet ingredients to the dry ones, mixing just until they are combined. Pour the batter into the prepared baking pan.

5. Bake until a knife inserted in the center comes out clean, about 45 minutes.

6. Cool in the pan for 10 minutes. Turn the loaf out of the pan and set on a baking rack to cool completely. This bread keeps, wrapped in foil, for 3 to 4 days.

OPTIONS: Use oregano or mint in place of the basil.

COOKING FOR TWO: This bread freezes well, so well you can put some of it away for future use.

sides and starches

tomato and blood orange salad

SERVES 4, 73 CALORIES, 3 GRAMS OF FAT PER SERVING.

The flavor of blood orange reminds some people of raspberries. While they grow in California, the blood oranges that come from Sicily between December and May are considered the best. Anthocyanins, which stain blood oranges red, along with the lycopene in tomatoes and curcumin in the spices of this salad are all cancer-preventative phytochemicals. This salad is simple to prepare. Its lush, Moroccan flavor will make you want to serve it regularly. Use navel oranges when you can't get blood oranges.

2 large, ripe tomatoes, cut in ¾-inch slices
2 blood or navel oranges, peeled and cut in ½-inch slices
2 tablespoons thinly sliced red onion crescents
Juice of ½ lime
2 teaspoons extra-virgin olive oil
¼ teaspoon ground cumin
Pinch ground cinnamon
Salt and freshly ground pepper to taste

1. Alternate the slices of tomato and oranges on a serving plate, arranging them in rows or in a ring. Sprinkle the onion crescents over the sliced tomato and orange.

2. In a small bowl, combine the lime juice, oil, cumin, and cinnamon. Add any juices that may have collected from the sliced oranges and tomatoes. Season to taste with salt and pepper.

3. Pour the dressing over the salad. Cover with plastic and set aside for 20 minutes to allow the flavors to blend. Serve immediately.

OPTIONS: Segment the oranges instead of slicing them. Arrange over the sliced tomatoes, along with sliced radishes in place of the onion. Use the same dressing.

Chop up leftovers and combine with diced roast chicken to make a salad. COOKING FOR TWO: Use just one tomato and one orange. Use extra dressing over a green salad or drizzle over steamed vegetables, such as green beans.

sweet 'n' sour onions

SERVES 4–6, ABOUT 43 CALORIES, 2 GRAMS OF FAT PER SERVING.

Italians call these piquant onions *agro-dolce*, or sharp and sweet. They are a perfect accompaniment with roast chicken or baked fish. Their creamy texture also makes them excellent stuffed into a baked potato, a comforting combination that is a great way of boosting your vitamin C consumption for the day.

2 teaspoons extra-virgin olive oil
2 large (2 pounds) Spanish onions, thinly sliced
1 tablespoon honey
1 tablespoon white wine vinegar
1 tablespoon fresh thyme leaves, or ¼ teaspoon dried
Salt and freshly ground pepper to taste

1. Heat the oil in a large, heavy skillet over medium-high heat. Stir in the onions until coated with the oil. Reduce the heat to medium and cook until the onions are softened and moist, stirring occasionally, about 15 minutes. Do not allow the onions to brown.

2. Return the heat to medium-high and cook, stirring often, until the onions start to color. Mix in the honey, vinegar, and thyme. Add salt and pepper to taste. Cook until the onions are very limp and golden in color, about 5 minutes, stirring often to prevent them from browning. Serve warm or at room temperature. These onions keep 2 to 3 days in the refrigerator, in a tightly covered container.

OPTIONS: Use red wine vinegar or lemon juice in place of the white wine vinegar. In place of the vinegar and thyme, use chicken broth and ½ teaspoon paprika.

COOKING FOR TWO: Since this condiment keeps well, use it to dress up simple meals over a few days.

braised fennel and tomatoes

SERVES 4, 61 CALORIES, 2 GRAMS OF FAT PER SERVING.

Fennel has a licorice taste that harmonizes perfectly with the tart-sweet flavor of tomatoes. This colorful dish works well even when tomatoes are not at their best. In fact, you can replace fresh ones with diced canned tomatoes if you wish. Serve this dish warm, as a vegetable, or at room temperature as part of an antipasto.

    1 pound bulb fennel
    4 large plum tomatoes
    ½ teaspoon salt
    Freshly ground pepper to taste
    ¼ cup vegetable broth, chicken broth, or water
    1 teaspoon extra-virgin olive oil

1. Preheat the oven to 375°F. Spray an 8-inch baking dish with nonstick cooking spray. Set aside.

2. Trim the fennel, cutting off the top stalks and feathery greens and about ¼-inch of the woody bottom part. Pull off and discard the tough outer layer. Halve the fennel vertically, cutting it across the wider way. Cut each half vertically into 5 to 6 wedges. Set aside.

3. Cut the top and bottom tip off the tomatoes. Cut each tomato into 3 to 4 thick slices, about ¾-inch each.

4. Arrange the fennel in two overlapping rows to cover the bottom of the baking dish. Sprinkle with half the salt and a few grinds of pepper. Arrange the sliced tomatoes in one layer over the fennel. Season with the remaining salt and pepper. Pour in the vegetable broth, chicken broth, or water. Drizzle the oil over the tomatoes. Cover the dish with foil.

5. Bake 45 minutes, until the fennel is tender when pierced with a knife. Serve warm, not hot, or at room temperature.

OPTIONS: When the vegetables are tender, sprinkle with 2 tablespoons grated Parmesan cheese and bake, uncovered, 5 minutes more.
Combine 1 tablespoon grated Parmesan cheese with 1 tablespoon bread crumbs and bake until the crumbs are lightly browned, 8-10 minutes.

COOKING FOR TWO: This dish makes delicious leftovers. It is even better the next day. Or you can use only half the fennel and 2 tomatoes, cooking them in a small baking dish. Use the remaining fennel in a salad or as crudités.

garlic greens

SERVES 4, 106 CALORIES, 4 GRAMS OF FAT PER SERVING.

A generous amount of garlic gives these hearty greens sensational flavor. If the amount of greens called for seems tremendous, remember they cook down to a fraction of their raw volume. Use all four kinds of greens or vary the combination to your taste and according to what is available, keeping in mind that spinach and kale are more tender and sweeter than collards or broccoli rape. Good on their own, these greens are outstanding served as a topping over Oven-Baked Polenta (page 278).

    1   tablespoon extra-virgin olive oil
    1   small leek, white part only, sliced, ¾ cup
    3   scallions, chopped, green and white parts, ½ cup
    2   large cloves garlic, minced, 1 tablespoon
    3   cups chopped kale
    3   cups chopped broccoli rape
    2   cups collards, cut in ½-inch ribbons
    3   cups fresh spinach or 1 10-ounce package frozen, defrosted
    1   cup chicken broth
    Salt and freshly ground pepper to taste

1. Heat the oil in a large, heavy skillet over medium-high heat. Add the leek, scallions, and garlic. Sauté until the leeks are limp, about 4 minutes.

2. Add the kale, broccoli rape, and collards, stirring until they are wilted. Mix in the spinach. Add the chicken broth and simmer until the greens are tender, about 15 minutes, stirring occasionally. Season to taste with salt and pepper. Serve as a vegetable, over pasta, or on polenta.

OPTIONS: Mix a 12-ounce can of cannellini beans into the cooked greens; heat and serve as a meatless main dish.

COOKING FOR TWO: Leftover greens keep 2 to 3 days. They can be finely chopped and added to soups or stews.

braised red cabbage

SERVES 4, 128 CALORIES, 2 GRAMS OF FAT PER SERVING

The spices in this dish perfume the house as it cooks. They also provide important protection against possible cancers, because of the antioxidants they contain. This dish is even better reheated, so think asbout making it a day ahead, while you prepare another meal. Serve with Bronzed Pork Medallions (page 248).

- 1 teaspoon unsalted butter, or canola oil
- ½ medium head (about 6 cups) red cabbage, cored, quartered, and cut in ½-inch strips
- ½ large red onion (about 2 cups) thinly sliced
- 1 Granny Smith apple, peeled, cored, and thinly sliced
- 1 teaspoon ground cumin
- 1 teaspoon chopped rosemary, or ½ teaspoon dried
- ¼ teaspoon ground allspice
- ½ teaspoon salt
- 1 cup cranberry-raspberry juice blend

1. In a large, nonstick skillet, heat the butter or oil over medium-high heat. Stir in the cabbage and onion until they are coated with the butter. Cook, stirring often, until the cabbage is wilted and the onion is limp, about 15 minutes.

2. Stir in the apple, cumin, rosemary, allspice, and salt. Add the juice. Cover tightly and simmer over medium heat until the cabbage is soft, 35 to 40 minutes, reducing the heat, if necessary. Cool to room temperature. Reheat before serving.

OPTIONS: Add some cubed tofu and turn this into a meatless main dish, garnished with some chopped dill.

COOKING FOR TWO: This cabbage goes well served the next day with cold roast chicken or turkey.

acorn squash stuffed with wild rice

SERVES 4, 129 CALORIES, LESS THAN 1 GRAM OF FAT PER SERVING.

Squash is a wonderful, healthful vegetable too often missing from the american table. Ths delicious dish uses the sweetness of apples and the slightly exotic taste of wild rice to make a squash dish that will have them asking for seconds.

    2 small acorn squash, about 4-inches long
    2 tablespoons dried cranberries
    ¼ cup apple juice (optional)
    1 large portobello mushroom, chopped, about 1 cup
    1 medium shallot, minced, 1 tablespoon
    ½ Golden Delicious apple, peeled, cored and chopped
    1 cup cooked wild rice
    Salt and freshly ground pepper to taste

1. Preheat the oven to 375°F. Spray a baking sheet with cooking spray and set aside.

2. Halve the squash lengthwise. Scoop out and discard the seeds and stringy fibers. Place the squash, cut-side down, on the baking sheet. Bake until soft when the squash is pierced with a knife, about 35 minutes.

3. While the squash bakes, in a small bowl plump the cranberries in the apple juice, or in warm water. This takes about 20 minutes.

4. In a medium, nonstick skillet over medium-high heat, sauté the mushrooms with the shallots until the mushrooms let their liquid. Add the apple; continue cooking until the mushrooms brown and the apple is slightly soft. Pour the mixture into a large bowl.

5. Add the wild rice to the sautéed mushroom mixture. Drain the cranberries and chop them coarsely. Add them to the filling. Season the filling to taste with salt and pepper.

6. When the squash is done, spoon about ½ cup of the filling into the cavity of each half and serve.

OPTIONS: When you have leftover acorn or butternut squash, make this filling and mix in pieces of the cooked squash. Serve a grain side dish.

COOKING FOR TWO: When you have cooked wild rice, leftover from some other dish, use it to make half the recipe for the filling and stuff one squash.

okra with stewed tomatoes

SERVES 4, 51 CALORIES, 1 GRAM OF FAT PER SERVING.

Okra, a popular vegetable in the South, has become more familiar everywhere as interest in regional American food has grown. Even folks who call it "yuk-ra" like this dish because the okra is crisp, though it will get gummy if you let it sit for a while. An abundance of onion and flavorful stewed tomatoes complement the okra nicely.

    1 teaspoon olive oil
    ½ cup coarsely chopped Spanish onion
    1 cup (about ¼ pound) fresh okra, cut in ¾-inch pieces
    1 4½-ounce can stewed tomatoes
    Freshly ground pepper to taste

1. In a deep saucepan, heat the oil over medium-high heat. Sauté the onion until it softens, about 4 minutes. Add the okra and sauté 3 to 4 minutes, until it turns bright green.

2. Add the tomatoes, bring to a boil, reduce the heat, and simmer until the okra is crisp-tender, about 5 minutes. Season to taste with pepper. Serve immediately.

OPTIONS: Sauté a seeded, minced jalapeño pepper along with the onion.

COOKING FOR TWO: Halve the recipe, using a smaller can of stewed tomatoes.

potato gratin

SERVES 6, 161 CALORIES, 3 GRAMS OF FAT PER SERVING.

The full, cheesy flavor and creamy texture here prove you can cut the fat out of this popular dish with delicious results. If this seems a decadent choice, remember that the potatoes in this dish are a good source of vitamin C.

2   large russet potatoes, 1½ pounds
⅔ cup skim milk
⅓ cup evaporated skim milk
2   tablespoons flour
⅛ teaspoon grated nutmeg
½ teaspoon fresh thyme leaves, or ¼ dried
¾ teaspoon salt
Freshly ground pepper to taste
2   ounces shredded low-fat Swiss cheese

1. Preheat the oven to 350°F. Spray an 8-inch square baking dish with cooking spray.

2. Peel the potatoes and slice them as thinly as possible. Arrange a layer of them to cover the bottom of the baking dish.

3. In a small bowl, mix the milk and evaporated milk with the flour, nutmeg, and thyme. Mix in the salt and freshly ground pepper to taste.

4. Pour a quarter of the milk mixture over the potatoes. Sprinkle on a quarter of the cheese. Repeat these layers, ending with the cheese.

5. Bake, uncovered, until the potatoes are tender and the top is browned, about 30 minutes.

mashed yams and butternut squash

SERVES 4, 144 CALORIES, 2 GRAMS OF FAT PER SERVING.

Yams are one of the best ways to load up on beta-carotene. Mashing them with butternut sqauash makes them light and moist as well as adding carotenoids beyond the familiar "beta" kind. A bit of butter enriches this dish, bringing out the natural sweetness in both these bright vegetables. It also proves that everything is good in moderation.

    2 medium yams, peeled, cut in 2-inch chunks
    1 small butternut squash, peeled and seeded, cut in 1-inch cubes
    2 teaspoons unsalted butter
    Salt and freshly ground pepper to taste

1. In a large pot, steam the yams with the squash until they are both tender, about 20 minutes.

2. Transfer the vegetables to a large bowl. With a fork, coarsely mash them. Add the butter and continue mashing until it has melted. The vegetables should still have a bit of texture. Season to taste with salt and pepper. Serve immediately.

OPTIONS: Use yellow-skinned or white potatoes in place of the yams.

COOKING FOR TWO: Use half the amounts called for. The cooking time will not change much, if at all.

eggplant "gigot"

SERVES 4, 120 CALORIES, 3 GRAMS OF FAT PER SERVING.

In France, they often insert bits of garlic into a leg of lamb, or gigot, before roasting it. Doing this with an eggplant gives you the earthy marriage of roasted garlic and eggplant, all in one. Mashed together, the eggplant and garlic make a light dip to serve with pita chips. Or you can mix in chopped vegetables and serve the eggplant as a colorful salad.

 2 cloves garlic
 1 medium eggplant, 1 to 1¼ pounds
 2 teaspoons extra-virgin olive oil
 2 teaspoons fresh lemon juice
 Salt and freshly ground pepper to taste
 2 whole wheat pitas

1. Preheat the oven to 375°F.

2. Cut the garlic vertically into slivers ¼-inch thick. Cut the slivers crosswise in half.

3. With a paring knife, cut 2 vertical slits, each about ½-inch long and ½-inch deep, on one side of the eggplant. Make one slit about 3 inches below the other. Push a piece of garlic into each slit until it disappears or only the tip sticks out. If necessary, hold the slit open by reinserting the knife and pulling it to one side as you insert the garlic. Repeat this procedure until 10 to 14 pieces of garlic are embedded in the eggplant. It helps to stagger the placement of the slits, starting one pair closer to the top and the next closer to the bottom of the eggplant.

4. Cover a baking sheet with shallow sides with foil. Place the eggplant on it. Bake the eggplant 1 hour, until the skin feels leathery and the eggplant yields when pressed. Remove from the oven. Let the eggplant sit until it is cool enough to handle.

5. Place the eggplant in a medium bowl. Pull off the skin, using your fingers. With a knife, scrape any flesh clinging to the skin into the bowl. Cut off the top of the eggplant. Pour the brown juices from the baking sheet.

6. With a fork, chop and stir the eggplant until it is creamy but still lumpy. Mix in the oil and lemon juice. Season to taste with salt and pepper. Let the eggplant sit 30 minutes so the flavors can meld, or refrigerate until ready to serve. This eggplant keeps 2 to 3 days in the refrigerator.

7. Before serving, separate each pita into 2 rounds. Cut each round into 8 wedges and arrange on a baking sheet. Spray the wedges lightly with cooking spray. Bake in preheated 400°F-oven until the pita is crisp. Serve the eggplant, accompanied by the warm pita wedges.

OPTIONS: Mix ½ cup chopped tomato, green pepper, onion, or any combination of the three into the eggplant before serving. Drizzle with some of the Red Pepper Sauce from the recipe on page 241.

COOKING FOR TWO: There probably won't be leftovers, but if there are, they keep 2 to 3 days.

curried couscous salad

SERVES 6, 135 CALORIES, 3 GRAMS OF FAT PER SERVING.

A generous helping of curry powder gives zip to this pleasantly light salad, as well as adding a host of valuable phytochemicals. Making the grain with chicken broth adds deep flavor; vegetarians can use a vegetable broth. Serve this salad together with Tuna Waldorf Salad (page 270) and Carrot and Red Lentil Pâté (page 230) for a light meal or summer party buffet.

    1¼ cups Rich Chicken Stock (page 239)
    1 tablespoon curry powder
    1 tablespoon extra-virgin olive oil
    ¾ cup instant couscous
    ½ cup carrot, cut in ½-inch dice
    ½ cup Spanish onion, cut in ½-inch dice
    ½ cup tomato, seeded and cut in ½-inch dice
    ½ cup zucchini, cut in ½-inch dice
    ¼ cup dried currants
    2 tablespoons fresh lemon juice
    Salt and freshly ground pepper to taste

1. In a medium saucepan over medium-high heat, bring the chicken stock, curry powder, and 2 teaspoons of the oil to a boil. Stir in the couscous, reduce the heat, cover, and cook 1 minute. Remove from the heat and let the couscous sit, covered, 10 minutes.

2. With the tines of a fork, fluff the couscous and pour it into a large bowl. Stir the carrot, onion, tomato, zucchini, and currants into the warm couscous.

3. In a small bowl, combine the lemon juice and salt and pepper. Whisk in the remaining tablespoon of oil. Pour this dressing over the salad. Toss with a fork until all the ingredients are combined. Season to taste with salt. Serve warm or at room temperature.

OPTIONS: Mix in ½ cup canned chickpeas or ½ cup shredded cooked chicken breast.

COOKING FOR TWO: It is hard to make a small quantity of this salad, but it keeps for 2 to 3 days in the refrigerator.

radish and cucumber raita

MAKES 2 CUPS, SERVES 4, 79 CALORIES, LESS THAN 1 GRAM OF FAT PER SERVING.

Indians serve this is classic, cooling condiment with fiery curries. Enjoy it as a salad, along with Baked Tandoori Chicken (page 242), or present it with Curried Couscous Salad (page 293) for a light meal. Even people who don't like radishes will not mind them here. They will benefit from the vitamin C the radishes contain.

> 2 cups fat-free plain yogurt
> 1¼ cups coarsely shredded, peeled cucumber
> 1 cup coasely shredded red radishes
> 2 tablespoons finely chopped fresh mint
> 1 tablespoon finely chopped cilantro
> 1 tablespoon finely chopped fresh dill
> 2 teaspoons fresh lime juice
> Salt and freshly ground pepper to taste

1. Pour the yogurt into a yogurt-cheese maker or a sieve lined with cheese-cloth. Place in the refrigerator and let drain until the yogurt is reduced to about 1 cup, roughly 3 hours. Transfer the drained yogurt to a medium mixing bowl.

2. Squeeze as much water as possible from the cucumber. Add it to the yogurt. Add the radishes, mint, cilantro, and dill. Stir to combine them with the yogurt. Mix in the lime juice. Season to taste with salt and pepper. Serve immediately, or refrigerate up to 24 hours, tightly covered.

OPTIONS: Use the radishes or cucumber alone, or add only one of the fresh herbs. Add a small, minced clove of garlic.

COOKING FOR TWO: Try this as a spread on whole wheat toast for a snack or light meal and you will quickly use up any leftovers.

breakfast and brunch

buckwheat porridge

SERVES 4, 262 CALORIES, 4 GRAMS OF FAT PER SERVING.

If you have never eaten buckwheat, also known as kasha, this porridge is a great introduction. Be sure the box you buy contains the whole, toasted light brown groats. Most of the sweetening in this warming breakfast comes from the natural sugars in the apple and the milk. The yogurt adds calcium to this nutrient-rich breakfast, which is also high in energy.

> 1½ cups reduced-fat (2 percent) milk
> ¾ cup toasted whole buckwheat groats (kasha)
> ½ Gala or Fuji apple, grated
> ½ teaspoon ground cinnamon
> ⅛ teaspoon grated nutmeg
> 2 tablespoons maple syrup
> Pinch salt
> 2 cups plain low-fat yogurt
> ½ teaspoon vanilla, or to taste

1. In a large saucepan, combine the milk with 1½ cups water and bring to a boil.

2. Add the buckwheat, apple, cinnamon, nutmeg, maple syrup, and salt. Reduce the heat, cover tightly, and simmer until the buckwheat is soft and velvety, about 15 minutes. Remove from the heat and let the porridge sit, covered, for 5 minutes.

3. Meanwhile, mix the vanilla into the yogurt, to taste.

4. Divide the porridge among 4 bowls. Top each portion with a quarter of the yogurt, and serve.

OPTIONS: Add ¼ cup raisins, for a sweeter porridge. Use soy milk or apple juice in place of the milk.

COOKING FOR TWO: Reduce the total liquid to 2 cups and the buckwheat to ½ cup. Still use the half apple.

muesli

SERVES 3, 300 CALORIES, 5 GRAMS OF FAT PER SERVING.

1 cup rolled oats (not quick-cooking or instant)
¼ cup toasted wheat germ
1 tablespoon chopped hazelnuts or almonds
1 teaspoon unhulled sesame seeds
4 dried white figs, chopped, 2½ ounces
3 dried whole apricots, or 6 halves, chopped
½ apple, cored and not peeled
Pinch salt
1 cup fat-free vanilla yogurt

1. In a medium bowl, combine the oats, wheat germ, hazelnuts or almonds, sesame seeds, figs, and apricots.

2. Chop the apple, or shred it, and mix with the oats and other fruit. This can be done the night before.

3. A quarter- to a half-hour before you are ready to eat, mix the salt and yogurt into the mixture of oats and fruit and set aside until the oats are soft, 15–20 minutes. Portion the muesli into bowls and serve.

NOTE: In Europe, they commonly make this breakfast by stirring hot water into the oat mixture and letting it sit overnight, then add the yogurt in the morning just before serving.

savory stuffed french toast

SERVES 4, 280 CALORIES, 7 GRAMS OF FAT PER SERVING.

Creamy mozzarella, roasted eggplant, spinach, and colorful red peppers give this version of French toast a new twist. It freezes well, so make a double batch so there is some on hand for spur-of-the-moment meals. Reheat it in a toaster oven and you can take it on the road for a hearty, balanced breakfast to eat like a sandwich; after all, it is toast, eggs, and more—ready to go, all in one.

   8-ounce loaf semolina bread
   ½ cup 2-percent milk
   2 eggs, plus 1 white
   2 ounces reduced-fat mozzarella, shredded
   ¼ cup defrosted, squeezed-out frozen spinach
   4 ½-inch slices eggplant, roasted
   2 roasted red peppers

1. Slicing the bread diagonally, cut off and discard the ends. Cut the remaining bread into 4 thick slices. Place each slice cut-side down and make a slit along the side, cutting almost from the top through to the bottom crust, and taking care to leave the bread hinged together.

2. In a large bowl, beat together the milk and eggs. Set aside.

3. Spread about 1 teaspoon of the shredded cheese on the bottom of the pocket in each piece of bread. Cover with a quarter of the spinach, arranging it to cover the entire surface. Sprinkle on another teaspoon of the cheese. Cover this with the roasted eggplant, then the red pepper, trimming each so it just fits the bread. Top with the remaining cheese, making four stuffed sandwiches.

4. Gently place the filled bread into the egg mixture, one cut-side down. Soak 10 minutes, turn, and let soak 10 minutes on the other side.

5. Heat a medium, nonstick skillet very generously with cooking spray and place over medium-high heat. Arrange the 4 stuffed pieces of bread in the pan. Cook until browned, 4 to 5 minutes. Turn and brown the other side. Serve immediately.

chicken hash

SERVES 4, 207 CALORIES, 6 GRAMS OF FAT PER SERVING.

Chicken Hash has an elegant air that is perfect for a weekend brunch. Evaporated skim milk keeps down the fat calories here, while adding creamy richness. Browning this hash takes a few minutes; the flavor and crispness it adds are worth the time. Hash began as a way to use up leftovers. In this case, making an extra potato and cooking an additional chicken breast a day or two ahead will save time.

- 1 tablespoon canola oil
- ¾ cup finely chopped onion
- ¾ cup finely chopped mushrooms
- 1 large yellow-skinned or white potato, peeled
- 1 tablespoon flour
- ½ teaspoon poultry seasoning, or ¾ teaspoon dried thyme
- 2 cups cooked chicken breast (1 whole breast), cut in ¾-inch cubes
- ½ cup evaporated skim milk
- Salt and freshly ground pepper to taste

1. Boil or steam the potato. When cool, cut it into ½-inch cubes.

2. In a medium, nonstick skillet, heat the oil over medium-high heat. Add the onion, mushrooms and potatoes. Sauté until the onion is soft, about 8 minutes.

3. Stir in the flour until the vegetables are coated. Cook over medium heat for 2 minutes, stirring often. Take care not to let the flour color, reducing the heat, if necessary.

4. Add the poultry seasoning, chicken, and milk, salt, and pepper. Stir until the hash is creamy, about 1 minute. Pat it into a flat disk covering the pan. Cook until the bottom is nicely browned and crusty, about 10 minutes.

5. Slip the hash onto a large plate. Invert a second plate and place it over the hash. Flip the plates, so the browned side of the hash is on top. Slip the hash back into the pan and brown the second side, 8 to 10 minutes. Serve immediately.

OPTIONS: Use diced turkey in place of the chicken. Instead of mushrooms, add chopped red and green bell peppers.

COOKING FOR TWO: If you don't want leftovers, use a medium potato and half the amount of all the other ingredients in this recipe. Watch carefully as it cooks, as these smaller amounts will cook more quickly.

fruit-filled omelet

SERVES 2, 218 CALORIES, 6 GRAMS OF FAT PER SERVING.

There is always something festive about a fluffy, tender omelet. Here, adding a touch of citrus and sweetness turns it into an unexpected brunch dish. The fresh-fruit filling, lightly perfumed with vanilla, echoes the golden color of the eggs. It is punctuated with the flavor and bright color of strawberries, blueberries, and kiwi. Using equal amounts of whole eggs and egg whites adds lightness as well as reducing cholesterol.

FILLING:
½ banana, sliced
½ Golden Delicious or Gala apple, peeled, cored, and sliced
½ kiwi, peeled and sliced
½ peach or nectarine, sliced
½ cup sliced mango or canteloupe
¼ cup blueberries
3 to 4 strawberries, hulled and sliced
¼ teaspoon vanilla

OMELET:
2 eggs
2 egg whites
1 teaspoon extra-fine sugar
½ teaspoon grated lemon zest

1. In a medium bowl, combine the fruit. Add the vanilla and toss. Set aside.

2. In another bowl, whisk together the eggs and whites until well mixed. Add the sugar and lemon zest and whisk to blend.

3. Spray a medium, nonstick skillet generously with cooking spray. Place the pan over medium-high heat. Pour in the egg mixture. As the eggs set, with a fork or spatula keep lifting the edges of the omelet while tilting the pan so the liquid eggs flow out to the edges of the pan.

4. When the eggs are almost completely set, spoon the fruit from the bowl to cover the half of the omelet closest to the handle of the skillet. With the spatula, fold the omelet over the fruit. Quickly lift the pan and slip the folded omelet onto a serving plate. Cut the omelet in half and serve immediately.

hash brown potatoes with sweet peppers

SERVES 4, 187 CALORIES, 4 GRAMS OF FAT PER SERVING.

This dish can almost do double-duty as both a starch and a vegetable, thanks to all the colorful veggies it includes. A good nonstick pan with a tight-fitting lid is essential if you do not want the potatoes to stick to the pan or burn. The broth allows the potatoes to cook nicely in a minimum of oil.

    1 tablespoon canola oil
    4 medium red-skinned or white-skinned potatoes, peeled and
       cut in ½-inch dice
    1 small onion, finely chopped
    ½ medium green bell pepper, cut in ½-inch dice
    ½ medium red bell pepper, cut in ½-inch dice
    ½ yellow squash, halved and seeded, cut in ½-inch dice
    2 scallions, white part only, chopped
    ½ cup defatted chicken broth
       Salt and freshly ground pepper to taste
    2 tablespoons grated Parmesan cheese (optional)

1. Heat the oil in a large, nonstick skillet over medium-high heat. Add the potatoes, onion, and peppers and sauté until the onion is translucent, about 5 minutes, stirring often.

2. Mix in the squash and scallions. Add the chicken broth, salt, and pepper. Cover tightly and cook over medium heat for 5 minutes, until the potatoes are still slightly firm to the bite. Take care not to let the pan cook dry.

3. Uncover and cook 8 to 10 minutes, until all the liquid has evaporated and the potatoes are lightly browned. Stir the potatoes every 2 to 3 minutes so they color on all sides. The onions and scallions will also brown.

4. If desired, preheat the broiler. Spread the potatoes in a shallow pan in one layer. Sprinkle with the cheese. Place the potatoes under the broiler 2 to 3 minutes, until the cheese is browned and crusty. Serve immediately.

OPTIONS: If red peppers are too expensive, double the amount of green peppers and use red onion in place of the white to add color. Add or substitute other vegetables, including diced zucchini, carrots, chopped mushrooms, or leeks.

COOKING FOR TWO: This dish keeps well, so you have 2 to 3 days to use up any leftovers, but it's likely you will eat double portions of these potatoes and not have any left.

sunrise smoothie

2 10-OUNCE SERVINGS, 144 CALORIES, 2 GRAMS OF FAT PER SERVING.

The sunny hue and fruity flavor of this naturally sweet smoothie are a perfect wake-up call. Strawberries contribute ellagic acid and vitamin C, as well as a rosy outlook to this breakfast-in-a-glass. The banana adds complex carbohydrates and valuable minerals, including potassium.

1 medium banana
1 cup thawed frozen sliced strawberries
1 cup 1-percent milk
1 tablespoon orange juice concentrate
4 ice cubes

1. In a blender, combine the banana, strawberries, milk, and orange juice concentrate. Add 1 cup cold water and the ice cubes; process until the mixture is well blended. Divide evenly between two tall glasses. Drink immediately.

OPTIONS: Replace the milk with apple juice or soy milk if you avoid dairy products. Some soy milk is calcium-fortified, so you don't have to sacrifice this important mineral when you give up the cow juice.

whole wheat banana bread

MAKES 1 LOAF, ABOUT 10 SLICES, 206 CALORIES, 3 GRAMS
OF FAT PER SLICE.

This quick bread is made using bread flour. This gives it a lightness and makes it less sweet. Serve it for breakfast and snacks rather than as dessert. Whole wheat flour and oats add important fiber along with high energy nutrition to this pleasantly chewy bread.

TOPPING:
½ banana, chopped
½ cup rolled oats (not quick-cooking or instant)
¼ cup light brown sugar

Bread:
1 cup whole wheat flour
1 cup unbleached white bread flour
½ cup light brown sugar
2 teaspoons baking powder
¼ teaspoon salt
2 ripe medium bananas
2 eggs, lightly beaten
1 cup low-fat buttermilk
1 tablespoon canola oil

1. Preheat oven to 375°F. Spray a 9-inch x 5-inch x 2½-inch loaf pan with cooking spray.

2. In a small bowl, combine the chopped bananas, oats, and sugar for the topping. Set aside.

3. In a large bowl, whisk together the whole wheat flour, white bread flour, sugar, baking powder, and salt to combine them.

4. In a small bowl, mash the banana mixture; there should be 1 cup. Mix in the eggs, buttermilk, and oil.

5. Stir the wet ingredients into the dry ones, mixing just until they are combined. Pour the batter into the prepared pan. Sprinkle the topping evenly over the batter.

6. Bake until a knife inserted into the center comes out clean, 45 to 50 minutes. Do not worry if some bits of the topping get very dark.

7. Let the loaf rest in the pan ten minutes. Turn it out onto a baking rack and cool completely. Serve or wrap in foil and use later. This bread keeps 4 to 5 days, and freezes well.

OPTIONS: Omit the topping, if you wish. Add ¼ cup chopped walnuts. Spread with ricotta cheese and a sprinkling of cinnamon.

COOKING FOR TWO: This is a large loaf, so plan to freeze half or share it with a friend.

whole wheat currant scones

MAKES 8, 150 CALORIES, LESS THAN 1 GRAM OF FAT EACH.

Whole wheat adds nutty flavor, along with fiber and extra nutrients to these light and virtually fat-free scones. Lavish them with fruit butter (a fat-free spread), baked farmer cheese, or a dab of sweet butter. Enjoy these scones as soon as they come out of the oven.

    1 cup white all-purpose flour
    1 cup whole wheat flour
    4 teaspoons baking powder
    ½ teaspoon ground cardamom
    ⅛ teaspoon salt
    ¼ cup dried currants
    1 cup apple sauce (see Note next page)
    2 tablespoons sugar
    ¼ cup low-fat buttermilk

1. Preheat the oven to 375°F.

2. Sift the white and whole wheat flours, baking powder, cardamom, and salt together into a large bowl. Sprinkle the currants over the mixture.

3. In a small bowl, combine the applesauce, sugar, and buttermilk. Add to the dry ingredients and mix briskly to form a soft dough.

4. Drop the dough, ½ cup at a time, onto a baking sheet, spacing the scones 3 inches apart.

5. Bake until the scones are puffed and golden, 15 to 20 minutes. Serve hot.

NOTE: Use only sweetened applesauce. The sugar in it is necessary for moistness. Unsweetened applesauce produces scones that are rubbery.

OPTIONS: Use chopped dried sweet cherries or dates in place of the currants, and cinnamon in place of the cardamom.

COOKING FOR TWO: Make half the recipe.

<u>desserts</u>

cinnamon-raisin bread pudding

SERVES 6, 239 CALORIES, 4 GRAMS OF FAT PER SERVING.

Bananas, raisins, and dried currants give this dessert natural sweetness. Using sliced raisin bread helps you put this dish together in a snap. When buying the bread, check the label. Pick a loaf made without corn syrup or other extra sweetening.

8 slices cinnamon-raisin bread
¼ cup dried currants
2 teaspoons grated orange zest
2 bananas
1½ cups low-fat milk
½ cup lightly packed brown sugar
2 eggs
1 teaspoon vanilla
⅛ teaspoon ground nutmeg (see Note on next page)

1. Preheat the oven to 350°F. Prepare an 8-inch square baking dish with cooking spray.

2. Tear the bread slices each into 8 pieces and place in a large bowl. Add the currants and orange zest. Set aside.

3. In a blender, puree the bananas; there will be about 1 cup. Add the milk, sugar, eggs, vanilla, and a few gratings of nutmeg. Blend until well combined. Pour the banana mixture over the bread and mix with a rubber spatula to combine well.

4. Pour the bread mixture into the prepared baking dish. Let it sit for 15 minutes.

5. Bake the pudding until it is slightly puffed and a knife inserted into the center comes out clean, about 30 minutes. Let the pudding sit 30 minutes before serving, or cool until lukewarm. Cut into 6 pieces and serve.

NOTE: Freshly grated nutmeg has far more flavor than when it is bought already ground. Whole nutmeg keeps for years, and is worth buying at specialty food stores, along with the little grater made especially for grating it.

blueberry crumble

SERVES 6, 348 CALORIES, 9 GRAMS OF FAT PER SERVING.

The rich topping on this juicy crumble proves how a little butter can go a long way. The lavish amount of blueberries makes this dessert so succulent that the filling is almost a light pudding. Using a minimal amount of sugar lets the flavor of the fruit shine through.

FILLING:
6 cups fresh or frozen blueberries
½ cup lightly packed brown sugar
3 tablespoons flour
2 teaspoons lemon juice

TOPPING:
¾ cup rolled oats (not quick-cooking or instant)
½ cup all-purpose white flour
¼ cup whole wheat flour
½ cup dark brown sugar
1 teaspoon ground cinnamon
4 tablespoons cold, unsalted butter, cut in small pieces

1. Preheat the oven to 375°F.

2. For the filling: Place the blueberries in a large bowl. Add the sugar and flour, and toss with your hands to combine. Place the mixture in an 8-inch square baking dish and sprinkle with the lemon juice.

3. For the topping: In a large bowl, combine the oats and the white and

whole wheat flours, sugar, and cinnamon, using your hands or a fork to blend them. Work in the butter, using a fork or the tips of your fingers, until it is evenly distributed in the topping. Sprinkle the topping evenly over the filling.

4. Bake the crumble for 30 minutes, until the fruit is bubbling and the topping is lightly browned. Let it sit 20 minutes, then serve warm.

honey crepes with apple filling

MAKES 6, 166 CALORIES, 3 GRAMS OF FAT PER SERVING.

For a winter dinner party, this dessert manages to be both elegant and cozy. The crepes are as light as those including egg yolks and full-fat milk. Using apple juice concentrate and honey in the filling provides natural sweetness that takes the edge off the tartness of the fruit.

CREPES:
½ cup reduced-fat (2 percent) milk, plus extra for thinning batter, if needed
½ cup flour
1 tablespoon canola oil
2 egg whites
2 teaspoons honey

FILLING:
2 Granny Smith apples, peeled, cored, and cut into thin slices
2 tablespoons honey
½ cup frozen apple juice concentrate, defrosted
1 tablespoon lemon juice
1 teaspoon lemon zest
¼ teaspoon ground ginger

GARNISH:
Confectioners' sugar
2 tablespoons honey
2 tablespoons chopped pecans

1. To make the crepes, whisk the milk and flour together. Whisk in the oil, then the egg whites. Mix in the honey. Refrigerate the batter for at least 1 hour before using, up to 24 hours. The batter should have the texture of heavy cream. If it gets too thick, add milk, a tablespoon at a time, until it is the right consistency.

2. Heat a nonstick skillet, preferably a shallow one with rounded sides, over medium-high heat. Pour about ¼ cup of the crepe batter into the pan. Immediately tilt the pan, rotating it so the batter coats the bottom of the pan evenly. Cook until the crepe is set and the top looks dull, 3 to 4 minutes. Turn and cook until the second side is lightly browned in spots, about 2 minutes. Stack the crepes on a dish towel as they are cooked.

3. For the filling, place a large, nonstick skillet over medium-high heat. Add the apples, honey, apple juice concentrate, lemon juice, zest, and ginger. Stir until the apples are coated with this mixture. When the liquid in the pan starts to bubble, 3 to 4 minutes, cover and simmer 10 minutes. Uncover and set aside.

4. To assemble the crepes, place a crepe on a dessert plate, with the browned side down. Spoon a sixth of the apple filling across the center third of the crepe. Fold both sides over to cover the filling. Gently roll the filled crepe over. Sprinkle with Confectioners' sugar. Drizzle about ½ teaspoon of honey from the tines of a fork over the crepe. Sprinkle with 1 teaspoon of the pecans.

OPTIONS: Keep cooking the apple filling until it becomes applesauce. Sweeten it with some vanilla extract and spoon into the crepes.

COOKING FOR TWO: Make the entire crepe recipe and freeze the ones you do not use. (They freeze beautifully.) Make half the filling, using a large, shallow saucepan in place of the skillet.

strawberry pudding with blueberry sauce

SERVES 4, 313 CALORIES, LESS THAN ONE GRAM OF FAT PER SERVING.

A strawberry lover's delight, this colorful dessert is actually a version of old-fashioned cornstarch pudding. Yogurt adds creamy lightness without fat. Serve this pudding, layered with the sauce, in tall, stemmed glasses.

PUDDING:
1 pint strawberries
½ cup sugar
1 teaspoon grated lemon zest
2 teaspoons fresh lemon juice
⅓ cup cornstarch
1 cup nonfat strawberry yogurt

SAUCE:
½ pint blueberries
¼ cup apple juice concentrate
¼ cup sugar

1. Hull the berries. Cut into quarters and puree the strawberries in a blender. There will be about 1½ cups. Pour the pureed berries into a deep, heavy saucepan.

2. Add the sugar, lemon zest, and lemon juice to the berry puree. Add 1½ cups water.

3. In a small bowl, mix the cornstarch into ½ cup cold water until completely dissolved. Stir this mixture into the berry mixture in the pot.

4. Cook the berry-cornstarch mixture over medium-high heat, stirring constantly with a whisk, until dark "patches" begin to appear. Reduce the heat to medium and continue whisking until the mixture thickens, turns from pink to soft red, and comes to a boil. Pour immediately into a medium bowl.

5. Cover the pudding with a piece of plastic wrap to prevent a skin from forming. Cool to room temperature, then refrigerate until ready to serve.

6. For the syrup, in a medium saucepan combine the blueberries, apple juice concentrate, and sugar with ½ cup water. Cook over medium-high heat just until the berries soften, about 10 minutes, stirring occasionally. Set aside to cool.

7. Just before serving, stir the yogurt into the chilled strawberry mixture until they are well-combined and the pudding is creamy in texture. Divide among 4 serving bowls. Top with blueberry syrup and serve.

OPTIONS: Puree 1 cup fresh or frozen raspberries. Strain the puree to remove the seeds and add to the pureed strawberries in the pot. Use the same amount of all the other ingredients.

COOKING FOR TWO: Make the entire recipe and share with friends or keep the leftovers for the next day. Use extra syrup on pancakes or frozen dessert.

sweet potato pie

SERVES 10, 284 CALORIES, 6 GRAMS OF FAT PER SERVING.

Creamy sweet potatoes and a snappy, gingery crust make this a pie worth whipping up often. For the filling, use what are erroneously called "yams," but which are actually sweet potatoes. "Yams" usually cook up sweeter and more moist than the root we see billed as sweet potatoes at the store. The red-skinned Garnet and bronze-toned Jewel varieties are particularly good for making this deep, dark dessert. It is so packed with beta-carotene, fiber, potassium, and more, that you might occasionally sneak a piece in place of lunch without too much guilt. Baking the yams really brings out the most of their texture and flavor.

CRUST:
1 cup graham cracker crumbs
⅔ cup gingersnap crumbs
2 tablespoons canola oil

FILLING:
2 pounds (4 to 5 medium) sweet potatoes or yams
½ cup packed dark-brown sugar

¼ cup maple syrup
2 teaspoons grated orange zest
1 teaspoon cinnamon
¼ teaspoon grated nutmeg
¼ teaspoon ground cloves
¼ teaspoon of salt
3 eggs, plus 1 egg-white
½ cup evaporated skim milk

1. Preheat the oven to 350°F.

2. In a medium bowl, using a fork, mix together the graham crackers and gingersnap crumbs. Add the oil and blend with a fork until they are evenly mixed with the oil. Add 2 tablespoons water and blend until the mixture has the texture of moist meal.

3. Press the mixture into a 9-inch silver-colored pie plate. (Dark metal will cause the crust to brown too quickly.) Bake 10 minutes. The crust will be slightly firm to the touch; it will harden as it cools. Cool completely on a rack. This may be done 1 to 2 days ahead.

4. Increase the oven to 400°F. Bake the sweet potatoes until they are soft, 35 to 45 minutes. When the potatoes are cool enough to handle, peel and mash them with a fork. Measure 3 cups. Set what remains aside for another use. (This can be done a day ahead.)

5. Reduce the oven to 350° F.

6. For the filling, in a large bowl combine the yams with the sugar, syrup, orange zest, cinnamon, nutmeg, cloves, and salt, blending them with a fork. Mix in the eggs and egg white. Blend in the milk. Pour the filling into the prepared crust.

7. Bake the pie in the center of the oven for 45 minutes, until all but the center of the pie is set; the center will still be slightly soft. If necessary, cover the edges of the pie with aluminum foil during the last 15 minutes to prevent burning.

8. Cool the pie completely on a rack. This pie tastes best the next day, when the flavors have had time to meld. It keeps 2 to 3 days.

golden fruit salad

SERVES 6 TO 8, ABOUT 58 CALORIES, LESS THAN ONE GRAM OF FAT PER SERVING.

Fresh fruit salad is nutrient-rich and naturally sweet. Think of it for breakfast along with a slice of toast, perhaps topped with yogurt for dessert, or as a snack later in the day. When mangoes are in season, this glowing blend of fresh and dried fruit adds a new flavor twist to an old favorite.

1   medium mango
1   Gala or Golden Delicious apple, peeled, cored, and thinly sliced
½   Asian pear, peeled, cored, and thinly sliced
1   peach or nectarine, thinly sliced
½   cup red seedless grapes, halved
6   whole dried apricots or 9 halves, cut in ½-inch slivers
1   tablespoon, finely chopped, candied or preserved ginger
½   cup orange juice
½   teaspoon vanilla

1. To cube the mango, place it on the counter. Holding a knife horizontally, cut off one side of the mango, slicing as close to the pit as possible. Turn the fruit over and repeat to remove the other side. Hold one of the halves in the palm of your hand, skin-side down. Using the top of the knife, score it vertically and horizontally, making the cuts about ¾-inch apart and slicing the fruit so you feel the tip of the knife against the skin of the fruit. Grasp two opposite sides of the fruit between your thumb and fingers and turn the skin back so the scored squares stand out like a porcupine's quills. Holding the knife horizontally, carefully cut the cubes of mango at their base, separating them from the skin. Place the cubed fruit in a large serving bowl.

2. Add the apple, Asian pear, peach or nectarine, grapes, and apricots to the mango and toss gently to combine. Add the ginger, orange juice, and vanilla, then toss again.

3. Let the fruit salad sit 15 minutes, at room temperature, so the flavors can meld. Serve immediately or cover with plastic and refrigerate 3 to 4 hours. The fruit becomes mushy if left longer.

crunchy chocolate chip meringue cookies

SERVES 8, 302 CALORIES, 5 GRAMS OF FAT PER SERVING.

These light puffs conceal the surprise of crunchy oats and soft pools of chocolate. If you have a standard mixer, making these simple cookies is really a snap. Bake them on a dry day or they may not crisp properly. And don't tell anyone what a good source of fiber they are!

½ cup egg whites, about 4 large
1¾ cups sugar
2 teaspoons vanilla
¾ cups chocolate chips
1¼ cups rolled oats (not quick-cooking or instant)

1. Preheat the oven to 350°F.

2. In a deep bowl, using a hand mixer, beat the egg whites to soft peaks.

3. Gradually beat in the sugar and continue beating for 10 minutes. The mixture will be like grainy marshmallow.

4. Blend in the vanilla. Mix in the chocolate chips. Mix in the oats.

5. Cover a cookie sheet with aluminum foil. Drop the batter in heaping teaspoons onto the foil, leaving 1½ inches between cookies.

6. Bake for 20 minutes, until cookies are lightly browned and firm to the touch.

7. Slip the aluminum foil with the cookies onto a rack and cool completely. Peel the cookies gently from the foil. Store in an air-tight container.

melon in ginger-lime syrup

SERVES 4, 123 CALORIES, LESS THAN ONE GRAM OF FAT PER SERVING.

This dish works almost as well with bland, underripe melons as ones that are sweet and juicy. You can even use the precut melon sold at many stores. If you are serving company, make this fruit salad with melon balls. After the melon is eaten, save the syrup to flavor another fruit salad. This appealing dessert happens to be high in fiber.

    1-inch piece fresh ginger, peeled, cut into 4 slices
    2 strips lime zest, each 1 inch x ½ inch
    ¼ cup honey, preferably orange blossom or wild flower
    Juice of ½ lime, about 1 tablespoon
    2 cups cantaloupe, cut into 1-inch pieces
    2 cups honeydew melon
    ½ teaspoon grated lime zest

1. In a medium saucepan, combine the ginger, strips of lime zest, and honey with 1½ cups water. Bring the mixture to a boil over high heat. Reduce the heat and boil gently until the liquid is reduced by one-third, about 15 minutes. Set the syrup aside to cool to room temperature, or refrigerate until just cool. Remove pieces of ginger.

2. Place the melon and the lime zest in a medium bowl. Pour the cooled syrup over the fruit and let it sit in the syrup at room temperature for 15–30 minutes before serving. To make this dish ahead of time, refrigerate the melon in the syrup, in a tightly covered container, up to 12 hours. Serve cool or at room temperature.

OPTIONS: Add halved green and red grapes along with the canteloupe and honeydew melon.

COOKING FOR TWO: Use only 2 cups melon and half the syrup, saving the remaining syrup to use in the next 2—3 days, on fruit or in iced tea.

13

menus

There is no single food or diet plan that automatically results in lower cancer risk. As has been noted throughout this book, cancer prevention is the result of a wide range of things, from staying active to eating healthy, over long periods of time. Therefore, the menus offered here are not meant to be seen as a plan of action that must be followed for cancer prevention. There is no magic in the food selections presented here. But there is good nutrition, a wide variety of foods, and plenty of good things to enjoy.

These menus are presented as an illustration that eating for good health and lower cancer risk can and should be interesting, enjoyable, and easy to do. You need only take a quick look through the suggested menus to see the principles being followed. The suggested meals are rich in vegetables, fruits, and whole grains. Fat is limited and fish and poultry are emphasized over red meat. There's a clear emphasis on getting a variety of healthful foods into your meals.

Yes, you could slice a banana on a bowl of cereal every morning and be getting a fairly nutritious start to the day. But when you add the variety of half a grapefruit one day, some strawberries another, and cantaloupe the next, not only have you added a great many wonderful new tastes and flavors to your diet, but you've added an amazing mix of nutrients and phytochemicals— things that all add up to a healthier you.

The menu suggestions offered here were created to meet the dietary recommendations for cancer prevention presented in the expert panel report, *Food, Nutrition and the Prevention of Cancer: A Global Perspective.* Use these menus as inspiration, not as rules that must be followed. Create your own menus, for a day, a week, or a month. Choose dishes that emphasize less fat, but that provide a variety of fruits, vegetables, and whole-grain foods.

It's fun to do. And you don't need to be a nutritionist to do it well. Pick foods you enjoy, pick a wide variety, and follow the basics of healthy eating. It's really as simple as that.

Enjoy— both a healthier life and the foods that help you reach that goal.

week of menus for stopping cancer before it starts

monday

breakfast

Orange juice
Oatmeal with sliced banana
Whole grain toast with spread

lunch

Tuna Waldorf Salad
Rye-crisp
Fat-free lemon yogurt

dinner

Creole Stuffed Peppers
Sliced tomato and basil salad
Whole grain roll

snack

Blueberry Crumble

tuesday

breakfast

Half pink grapefruit
Sunrise Smoothie
Bran muffin

lunch

Turkey and Avocado Wrap
Quinoa Tabbouleh
Fresh pear

dinner

Eggplant "Gigot" on romaine lettuce
    with sliced cucumber and green
    pepper
Whole wheat spaghetti with
    sautéed cabbage and onions

snack

Whole Wheat Banana Bread

wednesday

breakfast

Tropical fruit juice

Seven-grain toast with fat-free ricotta cheese and apricot fruit spread

Sliced strawberries marinated in orange juice and vanilla

lunch

Split pea soup with croutons

Broccoli-Stuffed Baked Potato

Apple

Fig bars

dinner

Turkey Cutlets with Honey-Mustard Sauce

String beans

Carrots steamed in vegetable broth

Whole wheat dinner roll

Fruit salad

snack

Cinnamon-Raisin Bread Pudding

thursday

breakfast

Muesli with yogurt

Blueberry wheat muffin with spread

Cantaloupe wedge

lunch

Kale and White Bean Soup

Whole Wheat Bread with Fresh Herbs and hummous

Grapes

dinner

Sicilian Spaghetti with Swordfish*

Sliced fennel and orange salad

Garlic Greens

Whole-grain dinner roll

Crunchy Chocolate Chip Meringue Cookies

snack

Raspberries with yogurt

friday

breakfast

Orange juice
One egg, boiled or poached
Whole wheat bagel with fat-free
    chive cream cheese

lunch

Carrot sticks with Spicy Spinach
    Dip
Polenta Stew
Seven-grain bread

dinner

Stuffed Portobello Mushrooms
Collard greens cooked in chicken
    broth
Raisin walnut roll
Fruit compote

snack

Oatmeal cookies with milk

saturday

breakfast

Grapefruit juice
Buckwheat Porridge
Fresh blueberries
Whole wheat English muffin with
    spread

lunch

Chicken Fajita
Spinach salad with fat-free dressing
Red Bean and Rice Salad
Sliced orange and banana with
    cinnamon

dinner

Halibut with Garlic Mashed
    Potatoes
Steamed kale with lemon slices
Carrots cooked in vegetable broth
Poached pear with raspberry puree

snack

Rice pudding

sunday

brunch

Virgin Mary
Chicken Hash
Whole Wheat Currant Scones
    with apple butter
Golden Fruit Salad

snack

French Onion Soup
Carrot and Red Lentil Pâté on
    whole wheat pita triangles
Fresh peach

dinner

Black Bean Stew with Pineapple
Brown rice
Mashed Yams with Butternut
    Squash
Mixed greens salad with fat-free
    dressing

snack

Melon in Ginger-Lime Syrup

in closing

The bad news? Even if you've read every word of this book, followed every recommendation for healthier living offered here, and tried every recipe suggested for healthier eating, there's still no guarantee that cancer will never strike you.

The good news? Making all the changes suggested in this book, or a great many of them, or even just one or two, will make a difference—a positive, significant difference in the cancer risk you face throughout your life. Maybe not a guarantee of no cancer, but the best chance possible today for avoiding this disease.

When it comes to cancer prevention, we are still forced to speak in terms of statistics for large populations, rather than specifics for individuals. We still understand too little of the cancer process and of the biology of our own bodies to be able to offer each person a specific formula or set of instructions on what he or she should do to make sure cancer never strikes.

But from a statistical perspective, there is an awful lot of good news and a great deal that recommends taking action now. We know that if the majority of Americans followed the basic advice offered in this book we could see an astounding reduction in cancer incidence rates. Get everybody eating 5 or more servings of fruits and vegetables each day and overall cancer rates could decline by 20 percent! Convince all those same people to also watch their weight and become more physically active, and those cancer rates would be 30 to 40 percent lower! In the United States alone that adds up to 400,000 or more fewer cancer cases, each year.

Too often we've become dependent on waiting for science to find the answers to our problems. Too much air pollution from automobiles? We design more fuel-efficient cars that emit fewer pollutants. Not enough food to feed the world? We develop super-grains and intensive farming methods that can triple production from the same amount of farmland.

But when it comes to cancer, science up to this point has not been able to deliver a "magic bullet" that will either prevent or cure this disease. While we have made amazing progress in early detection and treatment for many forms of cancer, we are putting ourselves at unnecessary risk if we simply sit back and hope that modern medical science is going to find the cure-for-cancer answer anytime soon.

322

As has been described throughout this book, the reality is that today we already have enormous power within our reach to prevent the majority of the cancers we now face. But the key to using that power is in the realization that each of us must take responsibility and make changes in order to minimize our individual cancer risk.

Eating healthier, staying physically active, watching our weight, and not smoking. It's not a complicated recipe for good health, but it's one that can pay enormous dividends. Most importantly, these are actions that can be applied anytime in life, and to whatever degree we each find possible. It's never too late in life to make changes for better health and cancer prevention. And there are tremendous benefits that come with taking even small steps toward a healthier you. It doesn't have to be an all-or-nothing proposition. When you do any of the things recommended in this book for better health, whether it's something truly big and life-changing, or just a small adjustment in your daily routine, it's a step toward lower cancer risk, better overall health, and less risk for many other serious health problems as well.

It's easy to make excuses and to put off making changes, especially when there's nothing wrong with your health right now. But don't delay. Prevention isn't about fixing something that's already gone wrong. It's about taking action now to ensure that cancer isn't a diagnosis that you hear from your doctor sometime in the future.

Stopping Cancer Before It Starts is not simply the name for this book. It's the end result we want you to achieve—an end result that's well within your reach. Start taking action today to make cancer prevention a part of your life.

acknowledgments

When an organization such as the American Institute for Cancer Research undertakes a project like the production of this book, it requires a team effort and a high level of cooperation among a number of people. Several of them deserve special thanks for the work they did in making *Stopping Cancer Before It Starts* possible.

High on the list are the two writers primarily responsible for most of the words appearing on these pages. Stephen Stark, an experienced science writer, served as the primary author for the science and advice sections of *Stopping Cancer Before It Starts.* Dana Jacobi, a food writer, recipe developer, and cookbook author, developed the recipes and menus in this book. AICR staff members John Lough, Dr. Ritva Butrum, Melanie Polk, and Sara Purcell also deserve to be recognized for their special contributions to this project.

This project was made possible in large part due to the support of the board and senior executives of the American Institute for Cancer Research. Thanks go to board chairman Melvin Hutson, board members Lawrence Pratt, Susan Pepper, Peter McCarty, Jeffrey Bunn, and C. Frank Newell, as well as AICR Ppresident Marilyn Gentry and AICR executive vice president Kelly B. Browning.

The most important element in the creation of this book, however, was *Food, Nutrition and the Prevention of Cancer: A Global Perspective,* the landmark report of the Diet and Cancer Project of the American Institute for Cancer Research and the World Cancer Research Fund that is the basis for the material presented here. Geoffrey Cannon, Sue Deeley, and Deirdre McGinley of the World Cancer Research Fund staff deserve enormous credit for managing the often difficult four-year process that resulted in that groundbreaking international report.

That project succeeded thanks to the dedication of the scientists who served on the expert panel for the Diet and Cancer Project. The panel,

324

chaired by Professor John D. Potter of the Fred Hutchinson Cancer Center in Seattle, Washington, included Dr. Adolfo Chavez, National Institute of Nutrition, Mexico City, Mexico; Dr. Junshi Chen, Chinese Academy of Preventive Medicine, Bejing, China; Professor Anna Ferro-Luzzi, National Institute of Nutrition, Rome, Italy; Professor Tomio Hirohata, Nakamura University, Fukuoka City, Japan; Professor Philip James, The Rowett Research Institute, Aberdeen, Scotland; Dr. Fred F. Kadlubar, National Center for Toxicological Research, Jefferson, Arkansas; Dr. Festo Kavishe, UNICEF, Cambodia; Professor Laurence Kolonel, University of Hawaii, Honolulu, Hawaii; Professor Suminori Kono, Kyushu University, Fukuoka City, Japan; Dr. Kamala Krishnaswamy, National Institute of Nutrition, Hyderabad, India; Professor A. J. McMichael, London School of Hygiene and Tropical Medicine, London, England; Professor Sushma Palmer, Center for Communications, Health and the Environment, Washington, D.C.; Professor Lionel Poirier, National Center for Toxicological Research, Jefferson, Arkansas; Professor Walter Willett, Harvard School of Public Health, Boston, Massachusetts. Our appreciation also to Professor T. Colin Campbell, Cornell University, Ithaca, New York, AICR/WCRF senior science advisor.

AICR's appreciation also goes to the representatives of the international agencies who participated in the process of developing *Food, Nutrition and the Prevention of Cancer: A Global Perspective*. They include Dr. Peter Greenwald of the National Cancer Institute, Bethesda, Maryland; Dr. John Lupien and Mr. William Clay of the Food and Agriculture Organization of the United Nations, Rome, Italy; Dr. Mark Tsechkovski and Dr. Elizbet Helsing of the World Health Organization, Geneva, Switzerland; and Dr. Elio Riboli of the International Agency for Research on Cancer, Lyon, France. Our thanks also to the more than one hundred scientists and public policy experts who served as contributors and peer reviewers for *Food, Nutrition and the Prevention of Cancer: A Global Perspective*.

index

about the american institute
for cancer research

Cancer can be prevented. That belief has been the vision that has guided the research and education programs of the AICR since 1983, the institute's first year of operation. As the only national cancer charity focusing on the link between diet, nutrition, and cancer, AICR has become a national leader in diet, nutrition, and cancer prevention, and has seen its programs in cancer research and education grow at an astounding rate.

In the early 1980s, when the AICR began, only a very small percentage of cancer research dollars were targeted for diet, nutrition, and cancer research. AICR's research grant programs have changed that by providing tens of millions of dollars for cutting-edge research into diet, nutrition, and cancer. This research has not only fostered a growing body of scientific knowledge in the field, but also has helped attract talented new scientists and encouraged additional funding from many other sources.

Most recently, after more than four years of work with a panel of fifteen of the world's leading researchers in the diet and cancer field, in October 1997, AICR, with its UK affiliate, the World Cancer Research Fund, produced the first major international report on diet and cancer, *Food, Nutrition and the Prevention of Cancer: A Global Perspective.* The report received worldwide press coverage upon its release and will continue to have an effect on the war against cancer by helping to set new directions in cancer research, public health guidelines, and public health policy for many years to come.

Simple dietary changes could save tens of thousands of lives in this country each year. That fact is why the AICR not only supports innovative research to expand scientific understanding of the cancer process, but also provides nationally recognized educational efforts, including award-winning booklets, newsletters, and a toll-free nutrition hotline (1-800-843-8114), to take current research findings and make them available to consumers for effective cancer prevention today. Additional information about AICR is also available on the Internet through the AICR Web site at http://www.aicr.org.

AICR can be contacted directly by writing to American Institute for Cancer Research, 1759 R Street NW, Washington, DC 20009, by calling AICR's toll-free number, 1-800-843-8114, or by e-mail to aicrweb@aicr.org.